BEYONDCRAZY

BEYONDCRAZY

JOURNEYS THROUGH MENTAL ILLNESS

JULIA NUNES & SCOTT SIMMIE

M&S

Cloth edition published published 2002
Trade paperback edition published 2004

National Library of Canada Cataloguing in Publication

Nunes, Julia
Beyond crazy : journeys through mental illness / Julia Nunes and Scott Simmie.

ISBN 978-0-7710-8068-5 (bound).—ISBN 978-0-7710-8069-2 (pbk.)

1. Mentally ill–Canada–Biography. 2. Celebrities–Canada–Biography.
I. Simmie, Scott II. Title.

RA790.7.C3N86 2002   616.89'0092'271   C2002-902127-8

We acknowledge the financial support of the Government of Canada through the Book Publishing Industry Development Program and that of the Government of Ontario through the Ontario Media Development Corporation's Ontario Book Initiative. We further acknowledge the support of the Canada Council for the Arts and the Ontario Arts Council for our publishing program.

Typeset in Sabon by M&S, Toronto
Printed and bound in the United States of America

McClelland & Stewart,
a division of Random House of Canada Limited,
a Penguin Random House company

www.penguinrandomhouse.ca

4   5   6   23   22   21

CONTENTS

This book is dedicated in loving, living memory to Odell Simmie and Leona "Sim" Simmie. Brother and sister forever.

ACKNOWLEDGEMENTS

We've been lucky.

We have friends, family, and employers who all supported this work – and who kept prodding us at those inevitable moments when our enthusiasm waned.

First, we'd like to express our deepest appreciation to the *Toronto Star*. This is a paper that *cares* – and was gracious beyond the call of duty in granting leave for writing and compassionate reasons. Special and lasting thanks are due to publisher John Honderich, who was a patron of Scott's initial mental health series. That project has now been the catalyst for two books and one career change.

Others at *The Star* also deserve our thanks, including Colin MacKenzie, managing editor Mary Deanne Shears, and deputy managing editor Joe Hall. Several members of the Ottawa bureau were helpful in trying to track down a couple of very busy – and often elusive – interview subjects. Kudos to Tim Harper, Allan Thompson, and Jim Travers. Supportive colleagues/pals at the paper include Dianne Forsyth, Leslie Scrivener, Barbara Turnbull, Jim Rankin, and Michelle Shephard. You're all invited to the cabin. (But not all at once.)

Thanks, too, to the good folks at Discovery Channel who have patiently accepted Julia's many comings and goings through the course of this book and its predecessor.

Of course, we're very grateful to the wonderful team at McClelland & Stewart, starting with publisher Doug Gibson. Doug has shown great enthusiasm both for *The Last Taboo* and now for this project. These books, quite literally, would not exist without him.

If there were an Olympics for patience, our editor, Alex Schultz, would be sporting about seven gold medals. He was extremely understanding when we begged, repeatedly, for deadlines to be pushed to distant horizons. Alex is also a great editor, and we truly value and trust his judgment. (We'll have that other section you desperately need at the end of next month.)

A merci-beaucoup to our copy editor, Adam Levin, who went over this manuscript with a fine-tooth comb and a very sharp pencil. (If you find a spelling error, you'll know who to contact.) And a big thanks for the design work done by Terri Nimmo, who conceived the look of the book you're now holding.

We're also indebted to all the wonderful people who submitted stories we couldn't include here because of limits on space. Thank you for trusting us. Your words helped shape this work. It was a privilege to be reminded just how wonderfully complex, fallible, and resilient human beings are. Maybe there'll be a sequel.

Brenda Nunes (Julia's mom!) was indispensable in assisting us with this work, transcribing so many interviews it's a miracle her fingers still work. Other family members provided tremendous moral support and were polite enough that, when we said we still weren't finished, they didn't ask "Why not?" Thanks and love to Alex and Rose, Lois, and Lyle and Kathy Jo.

It's likely, if not probable, that some names that should appear here have been inadvertently left out. If so, please accept our apologies and know that your contribution made a difference.

INTRODUCTION

ᨴ

We met in hotel lobbies, in the back booths of diners, once even in the front seat of a car parked at a roadside. We are not spies or drug runners; all we trade are stories. But stigma is a powerful force, and when the subject is our own mental health, we often speak in whispers, in places where no one else can hear.

Here's the good news, though, and we believe in it strongly. Human stories are powerful too. Told with purpose and passion, they *do* make a difference. They can break down stigma. And we all need to hear them. We know that because several hundred people have told us so. In letters and e-mails and snippets of conversation, they have thanked us for sharing our personal stories in our first book, *The Last Taboo*.

We always knew that other peoples' experiences with mental illness and the mental health care system were at least as interesting and illuminating as our own. And from the quality of the profiles people wrote for *The Last Taboo* (which appeared between each chapter), we were *sure* there were plenty more fascinating stories out there.

So we set out to find them. On the final page of *The Last Taboo*, we asked people to write down their own stories and send them to us.

We placed ads in newspapers and mental health journals. And whenever we appeared on television, we encouraged people to contact us through our Web site.

The response was truly overwhelming. If ever proof were needed that mental disorders affect every single corner of this country, here it was. We heard from doctors, lawyers, teachers, church ministers, and students, to name just a few. We heard from people whose careers are thriving, and from others who are unemployed. Some were angry at the state of mental health services; others were grateful for the help they'd received. And some people were sharing true secrets, talking openly for the first time in their lives.

We wish we could have printed every word that reached us. We truly do believe that each story has its own inherent value. But faced with the prospect of a ten-ton, ten-thousand-page book, we began the daunting task of picking and choosing. It was, without doubt, the greatest challenge in writing this book.

The world of mental health is so diverse that we could not hope to cover every point along the spectrum. This book is not a scientific survey. But we can say that it reflects experiences and perspectives common to many Canadians – the same kind of scope we'd aimed for in *The Last Taboo*. We did, however, seem to receive a disproportionate number of submissions from people who'd had a rocky ride in the mental health system.

That skew is, perhaps, natural. A person who immediately finds an excellent psychiatrist or effective treatment might not think they have a story worth telling. It is, after all, the journey that makes things interesting; an uneventful stroll to the corner store doesn't make for quite as gripping a narrative as the time when you had to dodge a car. Then, too, the person who had the rockier ride might have more incentive to write, thinking of their story as a tool to effect change (and we hope they're right).

For whatever reason, there was a tilt of sorts in the missives that reached our mail bag – so, too, in the stories that reach you here. But we're happy to report another skew – a common theme that emerges throughout the book. Virtually everyone you'll meet here has found a way to move on with their lives. And they wanted us to know about that.

Putting pen to paper or speaking into a journalist's microphone – saying, *this happened to me, and it matters* – is liberating stuff. And that's true whether you're famous or not, whether you live on the streets or in a penthouse suite.

Which brings us to the other part of this book. Over the past year, we contacted a long list of well-known Canadians – performers, athletes, politicians, writers – and asked them to share their stories too. Plenty of them said no. But a refreshing number said yes. Their stories are an important part of the reality of mental illness today.

In the twenty-first century, we've seen a movie about a Nobel laureate with schizophrenia win an Oscar for Best Picture. We've seen a story about anorexia on the cover of *People* magazine. In the space of a few days, on CNN's *Larry King Live*, Connie Francis talked about her suicide attempt and electroconvulsive therapy (chuckling as she calmly stated "I was a lunatic") and a beautiful model described the depression that followed a knife attack.

As a society, we are finally starting to acknowledge that depression, panic, schizophrenia, bipolar disorder – whatever other name you want to put to what ails the mind and brain – is all around us. But there is still a long way to go towards true understanding and acceptance.

The stories in this book will, we hope, help a process already begun – a process that takes us beyond the stigma. *Beyond crazy.*

As we often say, there are really only eight kinds of people affected by mental disorder. It's a very small list, but we all know someone on it: someone's mother, daughter, sister, or wife; someone's father, brother, husband, or son.

In other words, people just like us. Just like you.

Two quick notes before we sign off. The first is that we respected all requests for anonymity, so you will see the occasional use of a pseudonym; we look forward to the day when no one feels such precautions necessary, but in the meantime, we understand why they're there. We also added one or two ourselves for legal reasons. The second is that you will encounter many opinions about various treatment options and approaches to caring for mental illness. Sometimes, specific medications are mentioned. Any opinions expressed are the personal beliefs of the contributors to this book and are not a substitute for professional advice.

CHAPTER 1 WHO'S AFFECTED

—*m*—

There's a saying you sometimes hear in the mental health world: Labels belong on soup cans, not people.

It's become popular because, unfortunately, we often forget this little piece of wisdom when it comes to the people who've been diagnosed with a mental disorder. Many of us are still quite willing to read only the label and assume we've got the person figured out.

And so someone who might be hearing voices in their head becomes viewed by others as "a schizophrenic." A person who quickly swings from highs to lows becomes "a rapid cycler." A young woman with food and body-image issues becomes "an anorexic." We define the person by the disorder, putting that label before all other attributes.

Curiously, this is not something we tend to do when the symptoms are purely physical. We wouldn't call someone a "canceric," even if they were ravaged by the disease. It's a double standard that Dr. Michael Myers, past president of the Canadian Psychiatric Association, pointed out during a recent address to psychiatrists.

"When we call someone a 'bulimic,' we are conveying, inviting, and reinforcing stigmatized and stereotypic images of someone with an illness – and a shameful one at that. For the individual and the family, that hurts."

It does more than hurt. It blinds us to the fact that everyone with a mental disorder is – first and foremost – a person. It isolates people, branding them as somehow different from the rest of us. And it ignores the very real truth that one in five people in North America, in any given year, will experience symptoms that could be classified as mental disorder.

So who are these people? Who makes up the one in five? Surely there's something that sets them apart from all of us *normal* folks. Truth is, mental disorder does not discriminate. You could be a famous athlete or a struggling student, an aspiring lawyer or a young mom.

Mind you, even *those* descriptions are labels, ones that quickly conjure up pre-packaged images, our own tidy internal stereotypes that may bear no relation to reality.

The six people you are about to meet have all, directly or indirectly, been very much affected by mental disorders. As you get to know them, to know more about the whole person, you'll find that the labels disappear.

And what you're left with – regardless of diagnosis – are people. People not really any different from the rest of us.

ELIZABETH MANLEY
Athlete

Elizabeth Manley scarcely remembers the greatest moment of her life, the one picture-perfect performance that is the dream of every athlete. "It's a complete blur," she says, laughing. "I don't remember a thing."

That's okay, because millions of figure skating fans remember for her. The date: February 27, 1988. The event: the first winter Olympic Games on Canadian soil. It was the moment Manley had been working towards since she was first laced into a pair of skates at the age of three.

Calgary's Saddledome was packed that night, but the buzz revolved around two other women: a beautiful East German and an American pre-med student. Somehow, Katarina Witt and Debi Thomas had chosen to perform to music from the same Bizet opera; the stage was set for the "Clash of the Carmens."

Manley, unlike the Carmens, had never stood on an Olympic or World podium. Going into the long program (the final segment of competition), Leapin' Liz, as she would later be nicknamed, was third and expected to stay there, at best. Yet the skater herself remained optimistic. "Miracles happen," she told reporters, "in the long program."

And that night, one did. The 5'0" Canadian, overcoming flu, fever, and ear infections, outskated *both* Carmens with a four-minute flurry of triple jumps, breathtaking spins, and rapid-fire footwork, winning the night and (due to figure skating's complex scoring system) missing gold by a fraction. In the final seconds of her skate, she could not hear her music, so loud were the cheers, so overpowering the emotions.

"Sensational," the *Los Angeles Times* raved. "Spectacular," cried the *Globe and Mail*. Liz "gobbled up the arena and leaped to glory," said the *Chicago Tribune*.

For many Canadians, the most enduring image of those Games will always belong to the tiny skater, in pink dress and white Stetson, overcome with joy while the arena shook to the sound of 22,000 pairs of boots stomping in unison. It was, for many, the very definition of an Olympic moment – the one they all *wanted* to remember.

Although that single night was a Cinderella story (a role she would later play in an Ice Capades extravaganza), Elizabeth Manley will assert that her life has been no fairy tale. "People put people like myself or the Wayne Gretzkys . . . up on a pedestal, and they think we have the perfect life. And you know what? It's not all roses. You go through the same everyday life problems as your neighbour."

For Manley, those "life problems" have run the gamut from clinical depression to compulsive dieting. Along the way, she has done battle with skating officials who've spun circles around her already shaky self-esteem. (At the depths of her depression, overweight and almost bald, she says she was even asked *not* to compete at the Canadian championships. She went anyway.) Throughout, she has kept performing, ever popular with fans who love her energy-on-ice style. In this regard, and although she'd laugh to hear it said, Manley bears a certain resemblance to Princess Diana: popular in spite of, perhaps even because of, the emotional vulnerabilities she chooses to share with the outside world.

Manley could so easily have taken her silver medal and, for public purposes at least, lived happily ever after. Instead, she wrote two revealing autobiographies, *Thumbs Up!: The Elizabeth Manley Story* and *As I Am: My Life After the Olympics*. As a volunteer spokes-person for the Canadian Mental Health Association for many years, she spoke openly about her insurgent mental health. "I think it brings people closer to me," she says, "and makes them realize, 'If it can happen to her, then I'm okay. Look at how she's been able to turn it around.' And that's what I was hoping to do for people – just give them a little bit of inspiration to move on with life."

For those same reasons, Elizabeth Manley has set aside time for a lengthy phone interview with us on a Sunday afternoon between shifts at the rink. She has just returned from a skating show in Kentucky, succumbed to a bad cold, and allowed a group of pre-teen skaters, including her own niece, to camp out at her house while they train with her over the Easter weekend. "It has," she admits, "been a pretty hectic schedule."

Manley moved to Florida in 2001 to start coaching and choreographing young hopefuls (aged eight to sixteen) at a large skating centre run by fellow-Canadian Kerry Leitch. "I like it very much," Manley enthuses. "The centre is wonderful, the weather's great, and the kids are very hard workers."

At thirty-five, it seems Elizabeth Manley has come full circle.

Almost twenty years ago, *she* was the young hard worker, having won bronze and silver at successive Canadian championships. But mixed results in international competitions, she says now, prompted both her coach and Canadian Figure Skating Association officials to conclude that she wasn't living up to her full potential. They convinced Manley's mother that a change was needed, and at seventeen, she was shipped off to Lake Placid, New York, to work with a former World champion skater-turned-coach.

"So many things happened. All of a sudden, my coach, who was like a father to me, just packed it in and said, 'You're moving, and you're going to another coach.' . . . Everything was decided and done for me."

In a new city, away from friends and family, Manley felt everything begin to spin out of control. All athletes live on a knife edge, and now Manley started to slip, from confidence to fear, from the promise of a strong finish to the certainty of abject failure. "Every day, I felt myself slipping a little further downhill," she wrote in *Thumbs Up!* "I had always been a fighter, but now I seemed to have lost all my spirit. I felt scared all the time."

Manley, who had always been outgoing, became increasingly reclusive. Training by morning, she spent afternoons in her room eating potato chips, watching soap operas, and avoiding her schoolwork. Aware of how much her mother had sacrificed to send her there, and worried about disappointing her new coach, she told no one about her growing unhappiness. The need to please was paramount, an issue she'd grapple with for much of her adult life. "I wouldn't admit that I was unhappy, or I wouldn't admit that I was sad or confused. . . . I was a perfect person to hold everything inside and not realize I was doing it. I never complained. I never expressed my feelings."

What she held back emotionally showed up physically. Her hair started falling out, clogging her shower drain and covering her pillow each morning. Despite an increasingly severe diet, she was gaining weight by the day. "I guess my body went through this whole physical change to kind of wake everybody up, to say, 'Something's going on with your daughter and you need to figure it out.' They started taking me to doctors, and nobody could diagnose it, nobody knew what was wrong with me."

By the time the Canadian championships rolled around that year, Elizabeth Manley was half-bald and more than twenty pounds over-weight. Amid the open stares and catty comments of her competitors, the rumours flew. Was she in chemotherapy? Taking drugs? To no one's sur-prise, Manley performed poorly, finishing fourth, and losing her place on the World team. She returned home to Ottawa utterly devastated.

There, a doctor finally diagnosed her. She had clinical depression and a condition called alopecia, brought on, she was told, by severe stress, and causing potentially permanent hair loss. In addition to regular scalp injections, he prescribed a change of environment. "I think for me it was a bit of a relief," Manley says. "I got to come back home, I got to go back to my school again, I got to be back around people I was close to, and it just brought everything back down to ground level again for me. I think I just wasn't ready to be sent away."

The hair loss, however, continued. Liz's mother scraped together money for a wig, but, to fit it properly, what little hair remained needed to be shaved off. Young Liz gawked at herself in the salon mirror, tears streaming down her face. "It wasn't until they actually shaved the rest of my hair off that I broke down. And then, everything just came all at once: my crying, saying . . . 'I'm not happy.'" That day she told her mother, who had supported her through eleven years of competitive skating, that she was quitting the sport. "I remember coming home and saying, 'Mom, I don't want to skate any more.'" Manley recalls being "just blown away by the fact that she was completely all right with it. . . . She completely let me make the decision."

Manley began seeing a sports psychologist and thinking about what had happened. "I spent a lot of time on my own, and realizing what I'd been going through, and how I could control it, and what I wanted to do with my life." She also spent a lot of time talking with her mother, forging a deep bond that still exists today. "She was my best friend, she was my therapist, she was the shoulder I cried on. . . . I remember sitting there with no hair and I remember I wouldn't leave the house. . . . She just completely kept an open mind, and she listened to me. She never interrupted me, she just let me talk it out."

While Manley hid out in Ottawa, friends – especially those within the figure-skating world – abandoned her in droves. "You'd be amazed. Close friends and supporters just turned their back on me, because I wasn't going to do anything in the sport." Yet she now sees those weeks spent at home as the biggest turning point of her career. She grew steadily stronger, and the future began to look a little less bleak.

"It was kind of like crawling up these steps and then having to take ten back and then re-evaluating, and then starting again. I think it was probably the best thing that happened to me."

Within four months, Manley's hair was growing back, and so was her desire to compete. An unexpected phone call led her back to the rink to meet with two top coaches from the United States. Peter and Sonya Dunfield had helped coach Dorothy Hamill to an Olympic medal, and – despite her rusty skating that day – they were sure they could do the same for Elizabeth Manley. They even moved to Ottawa to work with her. "I came back with a whole new attitude. I came back . . . because I wanted to skate, because I wanted to perform. . . . I realized I was actually doing it because I *loved* going into the rink every day."

Despite the opinions of the Canadian skating world – "'Oh, she's washed up,' and 'She's just a head case'; I used to hear that all the time" – Manley's skating continued to improve. In 1985, at nineteen, she won her first Canadian championship, and cracked the top ten in the world. The rest, as they say, is all hard work and history.

After her silver medal at the Olympics – and a quick trip to the World Championships, where she again finished second – everyone wanted a piece of Elizabeth Manley. She was not just a medallist but a marketable one with a bubbly personality and a megawatt smile. Overnight, she'd become a household name, receiving a phone call from the prime minister, keys to the City of Ottawa, and a reception in her honour at the governor general's mansion. In Ottawa, an Elizabeth Manley mural filled one wall of the Elizabeth Manley International Skating Centre, not too far from Elizabeth Manley Street. Some of the kids circling the ice wore Elizabeth Manley skates and sportswear; at home, they hugged their Elizabeth Manley dolls, much as Liz herself had once hugged an old teddy bear for comfort before competitions.

A steady stream of television specials, commercials and endorsements, and skating shows followed. The highlight of it all, for Manley, was the chance to skate with Ice Capades; she quickly signed on as a showcase act and then criss-crossed North America for three solid years.

The pace was gruelling. "I did 1,200 shows in twenty-one months. I was just on the schedule from hell." And, Manley soon discovered, in the glitzy world of skating extravaganzas, image was everything. And that meant being thin. "I no longer could look like an athlete. I had to look like a showgirl. . . . You know what? I'm five-feet-nothing and I've got muscle coming out my yin-yang. How thin and elongated can a five-foot muscle-girl look? Physically, I will *never* be a Twiggy, no matter how hard I try."

But try she did. With the rest of the skaters, Manley lined up for mandatory weekly weigh-ins; anyone exceeding their pre-assigned weight could be fined or even fired. Manley, whose weight had been scrutinized as an amateur, put herself on a strict diet, staying well clear of her set weight of 114 pounds. "Working with girls who were four and five inches taller than me, weighing in at 10 or 15 pounds less than me, that's when I thought, 'Obviously, I must be too heavy.' . . . I watched these girls just not eat, and I watched how thin they were, and I just got caught up in it too."

Diet pills, laxatives, even cocaine were commonly used on tour, Manley says, and eating disorders were common. Manley's drug of choice was coffee, up to twenty cups a day keeping her going through the next city, the next show. "Coffee satisfied my craving for food," she wrote in *As I Am*. "Besides, it seemed the sanest alternative, considering the other methods that many of the skaters were using to keep their weight down."

Soon, Manley's own weight was down to ninety-two pounds – twenty-two pounds less than her Olympic weight, and exactly what she'd weighed as a ten-year-old. The response? Compliments at every turn. "For the first time in my life, I was actually having people say I looked sexy, or I looked good. And I got caught up in it. I became obsessed with it, and I loved the comments. . . . It's amazing how people love thin people."

On the ice, however, she lacked the strength to complete her jumps. Emotionally, she suffered, too. She was constantly on edge. "I remember snapping a lot," she says. "I would break down and cry an awful lot at the silliest little things that would go wrong. . . . And if I didn't skate well, I'd just be a complete wreck."

Throughout her career, Manley had been plagued by rumours, the most hurtful one being that she'd slept with most of the Canadian hockey team in Calgary. Although low self-esteem had, over the years, led her into several unhealthy relationships, she says none were with Olympic hockey players. (While on tour, however, a long, destructively obsessive relationship with a cheating boyfriend would add to her agitated state of mind.)

Now, word was she had a serious drug problem. Even her faithful agent came to believe Manley's frayed nerves and tumbling weight were symptoms of an addiction. Around this time, her Ice Capades contract expired. Two weeks into a new touring show, she was summarily dismissed, told she was too "sick" to perform.

It was the start of another long period of reflection and recovery in her mother's home. "If I hadn't gone through the depression when I was younger," she says now, "I don't think I would ever have overcome those horrible rumours about me."

Eventually, she got back in triple-jumping form, leaving the bad relationship, eating more healthily, and returning to her Olympic weight. She read books about self-esteem in an effort to understand why she had always been plagued with insecurity and doubt, why she had let other people determine how she felt about herself.

Once again, her efforts were handsomely rewarded. Manley went on to win three World Cup Professional Championships, including one win over her sexy former Olympic rival, Katarina Witt.

The night before our phone conversation, Elizabeth Manley did something she hadn't thought to do in years. Looking for inspiration for her new choreographing work, she pulled out a videotape of her Olympic performance. Diet Coke in hand, she watched herself skate, getting caught up in the moment, feeling nervous all over again. "I don't think in twelve years that I've ever sat back and appreciated what I did. I think I've just been going and going and letting everybody tell me what to do and where to go. . . . I don't take enough time to sit back and say, 'It's okay, you've done good, Liz.'"

Such is life for Elizabeth Manley, Canada's only women's medallist in the past thirty years at the Games' showcase event, in the world's most popular women's sport.

She lives in the United States, she says, partly because she is considered unqualified to coach in Canada. Much as Manley loves coaching – learning from her own experiences, she uses positive reinforcement on her young students – she would love to skate more herself. A recent injury forced her to stop training and she gained some weight. Since recovering, she says ruefully, "I'm not getting a whole lot of work coming to me. . . . I'm still doing some triples, I'm skating every day, but because I left a bad taste in my last few appearances, it's kind of put me a little bit in the doghouse."

Manley has pulled herself from more than one doghouse before, but at thirty-five she knows her professional skating days are numbered. Now she finds herself preparing for the kind of life she's never really known, away from the spotlight at centre ice and all those cheering fans, away from the only place she's ever felt complete. "When you're out in the centre of the rink, you feel that no one can touch you," she explains. "No one can tell you what to do. It's all up to me . . . and with all the politics and the pressures and everything that goes into the skating world, it never comes out on the ice. So it's kind of like my safe haven."

Months after our interview, Elizabeth Manley is back in that haven – on tour with the likes of Elvis Stojko and Brian Orser. It's a farewell tour for another skating darling, Josée Chouinard, and on the Toronto stop, fans at the mammoth Air Canada Centre soak up the steady stream of strobe lights, rock music, and champions. When Manley's turn comes, she races towards the spotlight in a black cowboy hat, low-slung jeans, and a halter top with large sparkling letters that spell LIZ across her shoulders. With a swing of her hips and an overhead slap of her hands, she gets everyone clapping to the heavy drumbeat of "Music" by Madonna. And for the next few minutes, she skates with a fury, moon-walking, doing mid-air splits, tossing her hat onto the ice, spinning round it twice. Such is the magic of figure skating: one small woman on two thin blades can energize an entire arena. And she does. She falls on her first jump and opens up on another, but it doesn't matter.

When the music stops, Leapin' Liz lifts her arms towards the crowd and they respond with one of the loudest cheers of the night.

GOING PUBLIC

Celebrity "confessions" have become almost commonplace, selling millions of books, magazines, and newspapers. We like to know that all those household names are fallible; that yes, they have money, fame and glamour, but *inside* they're just like us. That doesn't mean that it's easy for a celebrity to go public, describing those worst moments of their lives, but the people quoted here have done so without harming their reputations. And that is a step forward for us all.

ROSIE O'DONNELL on depression: "So I have written it down, my dance with depression. It is scary to read it back to myself. To let it go out there into the world, this dark piece of me. I wrestle the loud voices in my head: 'Don't write that. . . . Keep it quiet, Roseann. . . . Who do you think you are?' – And the meek ones that echo in reply: 'Hold on. . . . Here we go.'"

– *Rosie* magazine, September 2001

GERI HALLIWELL on eating disorders and depression, written the night before her final audition for the Spice Girls: "I feel like a saturated flannel is covering my face, soaking into me. What the hell is going on? Why am I like this? I just want to wake up and feel my old self. I feel as though I'm getting on everyone's nerves — my sullen face, my sunken smile and my continual frown. I'm always on the brink of tears. It's crippling me, I can't move. I enjoy nothing. I'm just existing."   — Geri Halliwell, *If Only*, 1999

SHAYNE CORSON, Toronto Maple Leaf, on panic attacks: "It was like everything was coming down on me at once. I didn't want to be away from home; I didn't want to be in crowds. It fed on itself, you know? The more scared I got, the more guilty I felt about being scared — I wanted to be strong! But it was so hard to be strong. . . . It's the sort of thing you hear about . . . people having anxiety attacks and panic attacks, and you think it could never happen to you. But it does, and it takes over your life."
                    — *Sports Illustrated*, October 22, 2001

MARIE OSMOND on postpartum depression: "During my childhood and teen years, I was abused. . . . I have spent many prayerful hours contemplating whether or not to reveal this part of my history. I found that my answer is that I can't be truthful about my experience with PPD [postpartum depression] without being honest about all the contributing factors. . . . What I didn't realize until I went for help is that I had never forgiven myself. Some part of me still felt I was responsible, that I must have been doing something to cause it. Those feelings spread into the rest of my life. I think this is why, at 39, taken over by PPD, I still thought: 'What did I do wrong? I am in pain — and I deserve it.'"
                    — Marie Osmond, *Behind the Smile*, 2001

CARRIE FISHER on bipolar disorder: "I used to think I was a drug addict, pure and simple, just someone who could not stop taking drugs willfully. But it turns out I am severely manic-depressive. It's taken me 20 years and a mental breakdown to say these words. I have two moods. One is Roy, rollicking Roy, the wild ride of a mood. And Pam, sediment Pam, who stands on shore and sobs. Sometimes the tide is in, sometimes it's out. . . . I am mentally ill. I am not ashamed of that. I survived that; I'm still surviving it."
                    — *National Post*, February 10, 2001

WINONA RYDER on anxiety attacks: "The worst part of it was not being able to describe it — the overwhelming horror of the anxiety attacks — even to my own family, to the people closest to me. . . . My breathing would get labored; everything would start speeding up, and I'd get very scared. The closest I ever came to describing it was that feeling when you almost get in a car wreck and you swerve, and for a second there are needles in your head and needles in your body. It's that moment, but stretched out."

— *New York Times*, November 14, 1999

MIKE WALLACE on depression: "A depression takes over your life. It is an utterly irrational descent into something close to madness. You wake up in the morning and all you want to do is go back to sleep — but you can't get to sleep. You've taken sleeping pills to try to stay asleep the night before, and you're groggy. It's an incredible experience. You think about suicide. You think about what a worthless character you are. . . . As it turns out, I was not unusual; I wasn't even in that deep of a clinical depression. For what I was going through, that was hard to believe, but my doctor said, 'Mr. Wallace, I've seen a lot worse.'"

— *Playboy*, December 1996

PRINCESS DIANA on bulimia: "I had bulimia for a number of years. And that's like a secret disease. You inflict it upon yourself because your self-esteem is at a low ebb, and you don't think you're worthy or valuable. You fill your stomach up four or five times a day — some do it more — and it gives you a feeling of comfort. It's like having a pair of arms around you, but it's . . . temporary. Then you're disgusted at the bloatedness of your stomach, and then you bring it all up again. And it's a repetitive pattern which is very destructive to yourself. . . . It was a symptom of what was going on in my marriage. I was crying out for help, but giving the wrong signals, and people were using my bulimia as a coat on a hanger: they decided that was the problem — Diana was unstable."

— interview on the BBC program *Panorama*, November 20, 1995

ELTON JOHN on addictions and bulimia: "I was cocaine-addicted. I was an alcoholic. I had a sexual addiction. I was bulimic for six years. It was all through being paranoid about my weight but not able to stop eating. So in the end I'd gorge myself, then deliberately make myself sick. For breakfast I'd have an enormous fry-up, followed by 20 pots of Sainsbury's cockles and then a tub of Häagen-Dazs vanilla ice cream, so that I'd throw it all up again. I never stood still. I was always rushing, always thinking about the next thing. If I was eating a curry, I couldn't wait to throw it up so that I could have the next one."

— quoted in Philip Norman, *Sir Elton*, 2000

ROSEANNE BARR on multiple personality disorder and other struggles: "I survived my childhood by birthing many separate identities to stand in for one another in times of great stress and fear. Each one was created to do only one thing. Every day is a struggle to remember, to hold on, to choose to live. I am an overweight overachiever with a few dandy compulsive obsessive disorders and a little problem with self-mutilation. No, no, no — money doesn't make it better, nor success, nor even a happy marriage. Every day I teeter on the edge of a razor blade."   — Roseanne Barr, *My Lives*, 1994

ROD STEIGER on depression: "When you're depressed, it's as though this committee has taken over your mind, leaving you one depressing thought after the other. You don't shave, you don't shower, you don't brush your teeth. . . . You don't want to communicate. You don't care about anybody's opinion. If Jesus, Buddha, or the Little Prince came down and said, 'What are you doing? I command you to get up!' you'd say 'Fuck you. Who do you think you are? I don't want to get up.' So that's the self-pity part."

— quoted in Kathy Cronkite, *On the Edge of Darkness*, 1994

DREW BARRYMORE on addiction and depression: "Part of being an addict is involvement in the continuous search for the perfect antidote to pain. It's like a doctor treating an illness with a specific antibiotic. For some addicts it's booze. For others it's pills or heroin. You go through them all, knowing that something out there is going to make you feel good. . . . Coke was the right drug for me. Neat and quick, with no apparent after-effect, coke allowed me to soar above my depression and sadness, above all my problems. What I couldn't see is that it eventually makes you go crazy."

— Drew Barrymore, *Little Girl Lost*, 1990

BUZZ ALDRIN on depression: "My life was highly structured and . . . there had always existed a major goal of one sort or another. I had excelled academically, being at the top

> of the schools and classes I had attended during my life. Finally, there had been the most important goal of all, and it had been realized — I had gone to the moon. What to do next? What possible goal could I add now? There simply wasn't one, and without a goal I was like an inert ping-pong ball being batted about by the whims and motivations of others. I was suffering from what poets have described as the melancholy of all things done."
>
> — Buzz Aldrin, *Return to Earth*, 1973

DAVID REVILLE
Politician and Advocate

Imagine life as David Reville knows it. The sheer magnitude of change: from law student to psych ward resident, from plumber to politician and special advisor to the premier of Ontario.

If we wrote the screenplay, no one would believe it. "Too far-fetched," the Hollywood execs would say. And they'd be right. But knowing this story to be true, we offer this condensed version of "The Life and Times of David Reville."

Main Character: At fifty-eight, with thick silver hair, sizeable moustache, and discerning blue eyes, he looks, his daughter has told him, like a chief of police. Yet the man is too rumpled, his smile too habitual, for that. Plus he has a really dirty laugh – the deep, rattling laugh of a pack-a-day smoker. Still, the guy has *presence*, and a suffer-no-fools countenance that's almost intimidating. "I kind of fancy myself as a guy with a wrench in one hand and a brief I've written in the other," he says, lighting up. "That's a fantasy I'd like to build about myself."

Setting: In an old brick building overlooking a freeway so crammed with bumper-to-bumper traffic it's dubbed the Don Valley Parking Lot by Toronto drivers, we find our protagonist's small corner office. The ceiling is a generous twenty feet up, but the room itself is a slender wedge with exposed pipes and small green-and-cream square tiles, evidence this was once a main-floor bathroom. Late afternoon sunshine pokes through the window at the far end of the wedge as Reville takes a final few two-fingered stabs at his ash-laden keyboard. Then he swings around in his chair and starts to tell his story. "It's very interesting," he says, "what I actually ended up doing with my life."

Act One: *Onto the Psych Ward*

On the racetrack and the football field, David Reville's high school years are a blur of activity. He plays Hamlet, presides over the glee club, is picked as school delegate to the United Nations, wins the Headmaster's Trophy. "I was," he acknowledges with a shrug, "a very hyperactive teenager."

At eighteen, he is dark-haired and handsome, as befits the son of a judge raised in a sturdy brick home by a well-to-do, solidly Conservative family in Southwestern Ontario. He's also leaving town, taking his overachieving self to the University of Toronto, where, within two years, he will gain early entrance to the country's most prestigious law school. At twenty, Bay Street is well within sight. There's a wedding, too – one that pleases both families.

Then the unexpected happens. David Reville fails his first year of law school. His father makes a few well-placed calls and secures a readmission. But the once-model student is rarely in the classroom. "I started hanging around a magistrate's court," he says, "as an alternative to sitting in class, listening to the same stuff again, and being embarrassed about being in the same year again. . . . I thought I would go and see what the law was all about."

In that big-city courtroom, a few blocks from the campus grounds, he discovers – and romanticizes – a world inhabited by prostitutes, petty thieves, and "low-level mafia types," all in need of legal representation, which our failed student is eager if not actually qualified to provide. "I started hanging out in what in those days was called The Tenderloin . . . where there were a lot of seedy all-night restaurants and strip joints. So I had what amounted to an office in one of these places, where I dispensed various kinds of – advice." That last word is said with an abashed laugh. "This was all going on in a sort of a spin."

The spin is fuelled, unbeknownst to anyone, by a rapidly developing mania. Soon David is hatching wild plans: insurance scams, movie-making, car theft. "I was operating as a con man, basically, and telling the wildest stories to people, who sort of nodded. I don't know what the hell they thought, but they handed over the keys to the kingdom. . . . My poor wife was quite surprised when the house of cards came tumbling down."

It all comes crashing down on a Christmas visit home to Brantford, where his parents find in his briefcase "a gun and odd financial records I had made, which to them seemed to be an indication of some kind of bad stuff going on. That was when they said to me, 'You've got to see a psychiatrist.'" David agrees, convinced the good doctor will declare him perfectly sane. "Except the psychiatrist didn't say that. He said, 'I think you'd better go to the hospital.'"

In a Toronto hospital, twenty-one-year-old David is told he has an "incurable mental illness" called manic depression. When he's released after four months of voluntary confinement, his life is a shambles. The young man who was, until recently, expected to represent *others* in court now awaits a criminal trial for car theft. His wife is not amused. "So things were not looking very good for me. So then I tried a suicide. And then I was committed."

David is sent to the Kingston Psychiatric Hospital where life quickly becomes Kafkaesque. He is placed on the geriatric ward, details of which he scribbles in an exercise book. "I walk past a long row of beds and into a large square room. The place smells strongly of urine. . . . In the room are about fifty men, most of whom are busy with various occupations – dozing, mumbling, sucking their toothless mouths in and out, and staring in a variety of attitudes: wistfully, stoically, blankly, demonically. . . . Lights begin to flash behind my eyes. Too much input: overload, overload, I'm shorting out."[*]

---

[*] Journal entries from *Shrink Resistant: The Struggle Against Psychiatry in Canada*, Bonnie Burstow & Don Weitz, eds.

For the next year and a half, the ex-law-student lives in this surreal world, which first confounds and later angers him with its utter absence of logic, method, or compassion.

"I didn't handle it very strategically," he says now. "I sort of acted up – acted out – in the hospital, which was mostly verbal acting out. And then I ran away once, but I didn't make it stick, which was foolish. . . . I basically turned myself in. And that left me being punished. They locked me up, and then they kind of threw away the key for a while. And then I really got depressed, and discouraged, and lost heart."

Transferred to a ward for violent patients, he's assigned to a prison-like room, a work crew, and occasional stints of solitary confinement. Throughout, he keeps writing. (On his twenty-third birthday, he notes that his parents send "socks, cigarettes, cookies. They think I'm at camp.") And somehow, he holds on to the notion that he will one day be released, unlike the lifers around him. "Most of those people, they were going to die there. Some of them had lost their language; they were gone. They were in comatose states. And whatever had happened to them had happened to them long ago."

In 1967, David Reville is – "by inertia, almost" – released. It's the Summer of Love, and yet he feels anything but free. He's lost his way, his ambition, all confidence. Also his wife, who left him six months into his hospital stay. "Now that I have nowhere to go, I can leave. But I'm already nowhere," he writes. "Hell of a place to build a new life. It's going to be a good trick."

Act Two: *Plumbing to Politics*

Back in Toronto, David Reville drifts. It's like being hit in the face with a two-by-four, lying flattened on the pavement, unable to stand up. "Things had been easy, and now they weren't easy. This nice elegant life was gone. . . . My whole notion of myself was gone."

So now he's an ex–psych patient working on a city cleanup crew. Mowing golf course fairways. Taking on a steady stream of entry-level clerical jobs. "Self-marginalizing," he calls it. "Part of it was my own sense of worthlessness, which I developed quite successfully while I was in hospital."

He gets married again, to a troubled young woman he'd met on the psych ward. They have two children and now there's a family to support. The young father fills in resumés, fudging the gaps, saying he'd been travelling. He's hired and let go, hired and let go. "They'd say 'Mr. Reville, you don't like it here, do you?' and I'd say, 'No, I don't.' And they'd say, 'Well, I think you'd be better off somewhere else.' And so I'd be gone."

Eventually, serendipitously, he's hired as a plumber's apprentice, "which is like a donkey or a horse or something." And back to school he goes, this time studying to be a plumber. To his surprise, he *likes* it. "I'd grown up in a family that had people come in to do stuff. . . . I had no mechanical experience or aptitude. So this was enough of a challenge; I really had to stretch myself to figure out how to do this."

Another world opens up, far removed from law school or The Tenderloin or the psych ward. Here, David Reville learns a marketable trade. From childhood, his father (now a self-employed labour arbitrator soon to be diagnosed with manic depression) had instilled in David the values of entrepreneurship. As a child, he'd fancied himself a businessman. And now, very quickly, he is one. He calls his company Alternative Plumbing.

His second wife splits; after several wild chases, he wins custody of the kids. And now he's repairing pipes in a downtown neighbourhood inhabited by well-intentioned parents who want the best for their families and are becoming community activists to ensure that happens. One of their leaders is a child-care worker named Cathy Jones, whom Reville meets and eventually marries. Her circle includes a few media types, and when *Canada AM* decides to air a segment on a new movie called *One Flew Over the Cuckoo's Nest*, David Reville is called in as a commentator.

Suddenly, he's on national television, a literate, lucid, self-described "crazy" who details the horrors of psych wards. "That got me rolling as a presentable and accessible commentator. Although I was *barely* presentable. I believe I decided to shave my beard off for the show, although my hair was still long and my moustache was Fu Manchu–ish, as would've been appropriate in the 1970s."

So now he's raising his son and daughter, with his wife, Cathy, in a middle-class neighbourhood. And soon he's caught up in the grassroots activism around him. He founds a neighbourhood parent-teacher organization. He chairs a community legal clinic. He canvasses for a left-wing mayoralty candidate. "And being an activist . . . is of course a wonderful antidote to self-loathing. . . . because the only qualification you need is that you're willing to do it. And if you put in some legwork and some skill, then you can do more of it."

Meanwhile, he pays the bills "doing the plumbing for all these middle-class people, city planners and whatnot, who have their little kid in Cathy's school. And eventually I get into positions of authority in the local electoral machines, so that by 1976 I'm on the election planning committees, and I'm learning what that's all about. And I'm meeting all the shakers and movers. And I have progressively more important roles. And in 1980, when there's a vacancy on the left in this ward . . . the sitting alderman says, 'Why don't you run?' So I do."

Getting elected, for a guy as sharp-minded and charming as David Reville, is "easy." His running mate, Gordon Cressy, has a name and a network, and "he basically allowed me to hop onto his big electoral machine, and off I went." Reville's psychiatric history is a "non-issue" – it's nothing he hides, nothing anyone thinks to ask about.

And so it is that scarcely a decade after he's been a resident of Psych Wards 6 and 8, David Reville becomes an alderman of Toronto Ward 7.

After five years on city council, the adjacent provincial riding opens up; the NDP incumbent has passed away. It is, Reville says, "sort of like God talking to me." And he needs to hear it, because life has again taken a turn for the worse.

After months of struggle, his fifteen-year-old son has killed himself. David Jr. had been wearing his distress in the form of full punk regalia – spiked leather jacket, fluorescent hair, chain attached to nose and ear. "My son was gonna be in trouble for a long time. He had a lot of trouble. And he just didn't make it out of adolescence, when it's troubling anyway." Describing this, David Reville's stream of energetic patter falters, and the smile, intrepid through talk of breakdowns and psych wards and his own suicide attempt, slips away. "He was a very talented person. . . . He was smart and handsome and full of beans. But he was full of pain. Oh man, he was full of pain."

Alarmed by his own mental anguish, Reville sees a psychiatrist and together they decide that he isn't crazy, "I was grieving." In the midst of all this, he somehow takes to the stump and wins his riding for the NDP. "People didn't have any clue that I was depressed, really. Then I went to Queen's Park, and found it pretty depressing there," he quips.

The newly minted member of provincial parliament decides to keep busy. He becomes a party whip, a House leader, health critic. "I got into it, and my depression went away, I think."

For the next five years, wherever he can, he puts mental health issues on the agenda. He writes amendments to the province's Mental Health Act, gets them passed in the legislature. He gives speeches across the province, telling anyone who cares to know about his time on the psych ward.

In the halls of Queen's Park, where the old boys' network thrives, David Reville fits in fine. It's a world, after all, for which he'd once been groomed. But life in the Opposition – the nitpicking, the posturing – starts to wear thin. In 1990, he decides to pack it in, start a consulting business. There's just this one brief stint as election campaign director, he tells himself, and then he's out of politics for good.

Once again, life has other plans for David Reville. The NDP shocks everyone (including its own leaders) by gaining a majority in the legislature and becoming – for the first time ever – the most powerful party in the most powerful province in the country.

The first few days post-election are – no pun intended – *crazy*. "There were just a few of us at Queen's Park being the government. There was no cabinet yet. And the phones were *melting down. Everybody* wanted to talk to you. I got to be in a version of *The West Wing* [TV show]. And that was exciting. And horrible."

Premier Bob Rae appoints David Reville his special advisor. Reville's first task is to break in the rookie MPPs who will be the government but have no experience of governing a province. Reville, of all people, will keep them busy and onside, because, as one press report noted at the time, "everybody likes David."

At forty-seven, David Reville has worked his way into a very elite inner circle, whispering in the ear of the premier. "I had," he acknowledges, "a scary amount of power."

Power – who has it, who doesn't – is an ongoing fascination. Small wonder, since he's one of few human beings to have lived at each of its extremes. "I became a New Democrat because I was mentally ill," he once told a Canadian Press reporter, making headlines with his trademark humour. "A lot of my politics were formed while I was in the hospital. Virtually every moment, I was reminded that some people have no control over their lives and that others have extraordinary power over men."

Act Three: *The Resolution (Life Today)*

In 1996, David Reville sets up shop. Hangs a sign – "David Reville & Associates" – on an otherwise unadorned steel door leading to the office that was once a bathroom. He's a consultant now. The same Toronto hospital he first entered as a psych patient now pays large amounts of money to receive his advice. "That," he says, with a mischievous smirk, "is *so* delicious."

He's in the boardroom, but also on the streets, where he applies what he now understands about power. And in essence it is this: Who has it, who doesn't, depends on "who gets which opportunity." His work today is about understanding, and overcoming, the unequal ways in which society doles out opportunities. "What you can do" – and the excitement in his voice is palpable – "is you can create some room for people to reconstruct themselves." And that "room" comes in the form of housing, education, jobs.

One example that touches him deeply: a sixty-two-year-old man who is learning to read. "He showed me an assignment that he was doing at school, and you think, Isn't this a fabulous thing? He's so beat-up, this guy. . . . He's been in jail, and he's been in hospitals, and he's been homeless. He's got no teeth. But he's happy, and he's so excited. And he's got *two* jobs now." Reville leans back in his chair, grinning broadly. "You can't beat that, right?"

Of all the labels David Reville has worn – golden boy, manic-depressive, MPP – the one he chooses for himself today is psychiatric survivor. It's a political statement, but also a symbol of the real bond he feels with others who've been where he's been. "My life is quite different from those of most survivors," he once wrote. "My connection is that I do know how it feels to be pushed around. And that I'm still afraid. Not about being crazy but about what they'll do to me if they catch me again."

Also, it's a statement about the course Reville's life has taken and the many forms of happenstance – good and bad – that have shaped that course. The time "in the joint," as he calls it, and "the poverty of not getting my act together for so long," and the "wrecked marriages and the tragedies in my life, which all have something to do with mental illness and the way it makes you act or feel."

All of which has led him here, to a place he seems to enjoy, an office far less grand than many in his past. Above his desk, he keeps a cherished photo of his granddaughter. On the walls, alongside the picture of himself with Prince Philip, there are framed awards from community agencies and thank-you notes from survivor groups. And when we've finished talking, as he turns the lock behind us on his way to another meeting, there's that sign on the door, the one he's earned for himself. The one that bears his own name.

At his seven-year-old granddaughter's urging, David Reville has now quit smoking.

PATRICIA VAN TIGHEM
Writer

What happened to Patricia Van Tighem one September morning could have happened to anyone. Patricia and her husband, Trevor – she a nurse, he a med student, both of them twenty-four – were hiking in the woods in the Rockies when a bear attacked. One minute Trevor was singing, the next a huge grizzly was on top of them, literally, attacking Trevor, chasing Patricia up a tree, dragging her back down to the ground. They would later learn that she was a mother bear protecting a carcass for her two cubs to eat. Small comfort.

Years later, Van Tighem described that day in chilling detail in her book, *The Bear's Embrace*. "A grizzly is chewing on my head," she wrote. "Crunch of my bones. Slurps. Heavy animal breathing. Thick animal smell. No pain. So fast. Jaws around my head. Not aggressive. Just chewing, like a dog with a bone."

Here, then, is the answer to that question anyone who's ever strolled through the woods has surely pondered. What would happen *if . . .* ? Van Tighem had the presence of mind to tweak the bear's nose, causing it to back off. Other hikers later helped them, bleeding and seriously injured, to safety.

Another question we all hope will remain hypothetical: How would I handle the aftermath of such a trauma? How does life go on once it has so very nearly ended? These are the questions that still tug at Patricia Van Tighem almost twenty years after the bear attack. "I never wanted to write a book simply about 'I was attacked by a bear' and entertain people with a sensational, gory story. I really resisted that," she says. "But when I started to write about surviving life after the bear . . . I thought this was actually about what scares all of us the most, [which] is no control, and a sense of powerlessness."

Van Tighem still struggles with those issues, struggles to live, in effect, with a sense of powerlessness. "We were just so happy [the morning of the attack] that it will always be a shock to me, literally, to have this thing come that fast and – *whack!* – in seconds to have everything be changed. It feels to me like that could happen with almost anything." Which is why she's travelled thousands of kilometres from her home in Nelson, B.C., and checked herself into the Homewood Health Centre in Guelph, Ontario, where she is undertaking a six-week in-patient program for posttraumatic stress disorder. "There's got to be a place," she says, "where I can learn to accept that I can't control things and still live in this world without constantly being on edge about what comes next."

As Van Tighem talks, at a picnic bench in what passes for a park in downtown Toronto, she smiles often, laughs (mostly at herself), and seems more at ease the longer we sit. At forty-four, she is youthful and bright and composed. This is the Patricia who's toured North America promoting her best-selling book, the Patricia who assures us she's up to an interview even while she's on a weekend pass from Homewood. This sunny Sunday in August is a good moment in a life traversed day by day, sometimes hour by hour.

On bad days, Van Tighem retreats to a dark room and "crashes," covering her head, unable to make contact with the outside world. She's convinced she does not deserve to live.

Sometimes, her two worlds collide, as they did when Oprah requested an interview. Most authors would keel over in gratitude, but *this* author was forced to decline, because she was, at the time, residing in a hospital psych ward.

Van Tighem has spent large chunks of time in hospital over the last two decades. Some thirty surgeries have helped reconstruct the entire left side of her face and skull, and removed infected screws, wires, and tissue. At the end of all that, she still suffers from recurring pain and infection. And she's still asked daily – in stores, restaurants, playgrounds – *what happened to your eye?* In fact, under the tidy, flesh-coloured patch she wears, there is no eye.

During her many stays on psychiatric wards, treatment has consisted of antidepressants, tranquilizers, mood stabilizers (which over time caused her to gain sixty pounds), and multiple rounds of ECT. At her worst, she says, she was "catatonically low," contemplating suicide, once attempting it. One year, she spent a full six months in psych wards in Vancouver and in her small town.

Yet all this makes Patricia Van Tighem's life sound far bleaker than it has been. Because between the hospital stays, she's also become a mother to four children (including twins, one of whom has Down syndrome), returned to nursing part-time, taken writing courses, founded a local support group for people with facial disfigurements, written *The Bear's Embrace*, helped Trevor design and build their new home, and held on to a marriage tested to its limits by all of the above.

"There was an article that said, 'In eighteen years their love has never faltered,' and I thought, Now there's crap! It's been enormously challenged." After the attack, Trevor, whose injuries were less severe and chronic, was thrilled to be alive, eager to get back to life as they'd known it, with hiking and camping and boating. At times, she says, he lost patience with Patricia's grief, sadness, and fear. And yet he did not lose his faith in her. "It amazes me that for years I was obese. I didn't look the same, I wasn't talking, really. I wasn't acting in a spouse role. . . . He just had this *blob*, is what I call myself then. . . . And he said through it all what sustained him was knowing who I was underneath it all, and holding onto that.

"That faith, to me, was such a gift, because I think I could have given up on myself a lot more if other people had as well."

Aside from Trevor, Van Tighem's mother, her close friends, and her four children have kept loving her, no matter what, and that has sustained her most of all. Children were "always essential" from the time she and Trevor met when they were both nineteen. "I'm grateful I have them. They're wonderful. They're really neat people. And I don't know what I'd be like without them. They're a big part of the definition of life for me." And they're the main reason she keeps up the fight. "I can't choose death," she says. "If there was nobody in the world who cared about me, I'd go ahead." Asked if she's sure about that, she laughs self-consciously. "Yeah, I would. But knowing how much it would hurt other people . . ."

For many years, doctors grappled with giving Van Tighem's turbulent emotions a diagnosis: first depression, then bipolar disorder, then a personality disorder. At the time of the bear attack, posttraumatic stress disorder (PTSD) had barely been named, and was associated mainly with war veterans. For more than a decade Patricia's symptoms went unrecognized: the recurring nightmares, extreme agitation, and ever-present fear of the unknown, which meant *everything*. "The bear attack was the quintessential sense of being held down and being powerless and not being able to do anything. But the rest of life became that way too. I never wondered why with the bear attack. I always just accepted it as a bad-luck scenario: in the wrong place at the wrong time," she says. "But I've asked why a lot around the depression, because I see it hurting my kids and Trevor. And I don't understand the why of that."

Hospital staff often seemed bothered by her inability to remain well, and she says she soon became known as a "difficult patient." Each time she re-entered hospital, she believed she'd failed as patient, mother, and wife. "A lot of what I've been dealing with is this realization of profound shame around the way I coped with it: I *needed* to be in and out of hospital. And I just warped it all into having done it all wrong." Asked what lies at the root of all that self-blame, she comes up with an unexpected answer. "There was a lot of religious dogma that I took to heart from the time I was tiny. When you put your hand on your chest in church and said, 'I am guilty' in Latin, I thought I was. I just incorporated that deep inside of me, and I was always guilty."

Then she says something truly astonishing – something that goes a long way to answering another of those hypothetical life-and-death questions we all pose. "I remember thinking at one point when the bear was chewing on my head and I [thought I] might die, that I might go to hell. And that shocked me afterwards, when I could think more coherently, that me, who tried to be a basically good person, could have that deep-held belief that I was that bad a person. . . . I rejected, after that, a lot of the [religious] dogma, and it left me with nothing. And I didn't realize how defining that was until it was gone."

So recovery, for Patricia Van Tighem, has been a process of rebuilding: definitions of self and of spirituality, concepts of faith, trust, hope, and, above all else, a notion of self-worth. The same questions we all grapple with, but writ large. And built against a hospital system that often reinforced the self-blame. She recalls being thrown into seclusion for the night on one occasion because she'd been unable to calm herself down. Being ordered angrily to *Stop crying!* when she awoke, sobbing, from yet another nightmare. She remembers arousing the anger of a nurse because she stopped at the front desk to ask for medication. "I remember the nurse snapping at me, 'Get your face out of here! I'm sick of seeing it around here! Go back to your room!' Yelling. And thinking, as I backed off, That would never have happened if I had been in to have my appendix out. The other nurses would've looked up in shock, the other patients would have. And yet nobody blinked an eye."

Van Tighem hastens to add that she also met with genuinely caring staff. But she has a theory about why she was so often treated differently on a psych ward than on a surgery ward. And it relates again to fear. "I come in on that ward in British Columbia. I'm a nurse, my husband's a doctor; they can relate right away. And I'm out of control. My life is out of control. My body is out of control. I wasn't somebody that they wanted to look like or act like. And I touched in them these potential places that could exist in them. 'That could be me.' And in the fear of it, there becomes rejection."

Which brings us back to the beginning of this story. What happened to Patricia Van Tighem could happen to anyone. That simple fact has brought her rejection, but also a new connection with the outside world. Her book has found readers across North America, and her readings inevitably end in standing ovations. Everyone seems to relate to her struggles, as well as to her courage. We all know, somewhere deep inside, that a bear attack (or a car accident, or a drive-by shooting, or even a mental illness) could strike at any time, testing our will to survive. But none of us knows how well we'd cope. All we can hope is that we'd find a way, and a reason or two, to carry on.

Patricia and Trevor separated soon after she returned home from Homewood.

MICHAEL WILSON
A Father's Story

Michael Wilson made the decision less than twenty-four hours after his son's death: he would not conceal Cameron's suicide. To hide the truth would be wrong, a betrayal of Wilson's own ideals – and a disservice to his son.

And so, in the middle of the night in late April, 1995, a grieving father climbed from his bed and began composing a eulogy for his child.

At the overflowing church, he told the many mourners – including former prime minister Brian Mulroney – that twenty-nine-year-old Cameron had been struggling with severe depression. That his son ended his life because of mental illness.

Three years later, the former federal finance minister made headlines when he spoke to a well-heeled audience at the Canadian Club in Toronto. The topic of his powerful address? The immense economic and personal cost of mental disorders in this country. There, too, he spoke of Cameron.

"He fought his illness. He was terribly frustrated by it," Wilson told the business crowd. "Those who suffer from depression usually want our help. They are lost and confused and, yes, they desperately need our help."

The sentiments were painfully heartfelt. But, as often seems the case when Wilson speaks publicly about mental health, the personal comments were brief – a snapshot within a wider message about suicide or stigma or the workplace or research. Cameron's story helps quickly put a face on the statistics, illustrating that those staggering numbers – some 3,500 suicides in Canada per year – represent real people.

Here, Michael Wilson makes a somewhat rare exception to speak at greater length about his son. And he does so for two simple reasons: the sixty-four-year-old is both an advocate and a father.

"Parents, I think, are probably in the best position of all to notice a behavioural change. And behavioural change is one of the fundamental signs of mental illness," he says. "If you see that your child is moving in one direction suddenly, is a different person, there's a reason for it. It doesn't just happen."

It's quite an assortment of adjectives that tumbles out when Cameron's two siblings begin describing how they remember him: athletic, argumentative, gregarious, confrontational, good-looking, protective, a partier, a *brother*.

He sounds, based on these reflections, very much like a guy's guy. An athlete who enjoyed working up a sweat in a good game of rugger. A pal who liked to knock back a few beers with his friends while watching hockey on television. A flirt who enjoyed trying to catch the eye of the prettiest woman at the bar. A chaperone who'd wrap a jealous arm around sister Lara when she started attending the same parties.

But perhaps the most consistent trait to emerge is one of a fiercely competitive young man, particularly when it came to his younger brother, Geoff. Born just 364 days apart, Cameron seemed to derive no small amount of his own self-worth by trying to outdo Geoff, whether it was on the hockey rink, in an argument, or in a wrestling match on the living-room floor. Geoff compares their spirited relationship to one of the more well-known rivalries in the NHL.

"It's just like when Tie Domi and [Donald] Brashear skate by each other – it doesn't take too much to drop the gloves," says Geoff. "It's true that much of our relationship was acrimonious and aggressive, but I think we both benefited from the competition."

Part of that conflict, says Geoff, may be related to the very different ways the two brothers dealt with their father's fame during their teenage years. When your dad is the federal minister of finance, he explains, there are some unwritten rules that go with the territory. You have to watch out for your *own* public image, and you're expected to learn the ins and outs of power, policies, politics. Geoff found this world fascinating, but suggests it did not necessarily hold the same appeal for Cameron.

"I think it kind of pissed him off a bit that he had to keep abreast of politics when he had no interest in doing so," says Geoff, who at thirty-six is VP and director of TD Asset Management. "And that's a

part of the stress that is probably most difficult for a child of somebody in the political arena."

Cameron preferred, instead, to throw himself head-first into sports,
excelling in hockey, football, and rugby during his high school years.
In those pursuits, he pushed himself to the very limits.

"He was a tough competitor," says his father. "He tried very hard,
worked very hard at it, and wasn't very forgiving on himself."

It was during his late teens and early twenties that outbursts of aggres-
sion, of raw anger, seemed to occur with greater frequency. Michael
Wilson saw it more than once on the hockey rink, but didn't quite know
what to make of it. Was it a phase, a rough patch? Or had Cameron
simply inherited a trait that Wilson himself admits to possessing?

"Some people would be surprised at me saying this, but his
[Cameron's] father had a temper, still has a temper," he says. "So he
may have picked up some of that temper from me and I thought maybe
he was suffering from the same sort of problem as I was."

Geoff, in retrospect, believes the problem had already moved
beyond anger management.

"One of my biggest concerns about Cameron through the late
teenage years is that the only way he really seemed to get any joy in
my presence was when he was putting me down. There was no joy of
success for a sibling, there was no joy in working towards a common
goal. The only joy was seeing me suffer or suffer a setback. Which was
very different from the relationship I had with Lara," he says.

Geoff recalls raising the topic with his parents and suggesting
in exasperation that Cameron "needs help." But, like many families
experiencing their first encounter with a mental disorder, it was easy
enough to think Cameron was merely having a rough time, that things
would get better.

And, for a time, they did. After attending Concordia University,
Cameron headed to England in 1990 to work in the financial field. He
spent eighteen months in an extensive training program with Baring
Brothers & Co. Ltd., a prestigious merchant bank. The strategy – earn
your chops in the City before returning to Canada and launching a
golden career – is a common one in this field. Cameron loved both

the job and the London nightlife, often staying out until two in the morning before being back at the office at seven.

And then, almost overnight, something changed. He awoke one morning feeling completely and utterly sapped, a sensation so strange and awful he would later describe it to his father as feeling like he "had razor blades in his mouth."

"He said after that he never felt right. After that, he would come home from work and he'd go straight to bed and sleep for two or three hours, have something to eat, and then go back to bed again. In other words, he just lost his energy, and we now know that that can be a sign of mental illness."

But no one knew that then. A doctor tested Cameron for mononucleosis with negative results. He saw other general practitioners on his return to Toronto in the summer of 1991, but no professional raised the possibility of a mental disorder.

"Maybe there's a message in there that doctors, GPs, have got to be more sensitive to picking up signs of a mental illness," says Wilson. "Or that GPs should be trained to ask more questions that relate to behaviour, as opposed to just saying, 'Oh, there's nothing wrong with you, kid!' Because there clearly was something wrong."

Despite his lack of energy and low mood, Cameron was no quitter. He landed a job as a trader at National Trust. But he had returned only to discover that Geoff's career was already well underway. Sister Lara believes it was very difficult on Cameron's self-esteem.

"Geoff had already established himself and got a reputation in that industry, and that industry is very close-knit," she says. "And I think Cameron was a little disappointed when he got back to Canada to see that he was known as 'Geoff's brother,' as opposed to Geoff being known as 'Cameron's brother.' I think that really bothered him, because he wanted to make a name for himself and separate himself from Geoff. And he had a real hard time doing that."

Whether this intense sibling rivalry was a seed for some of Cameron's troubles or merely exacerbated them will never be known. But during the years following his return from London, Cameron's outbursts – or at least the intensity of those outbursts – increased. The troubles spread to his job, where he was often on argumentative terms with his boss.

"There was an element of paranoia in this," says Wilson. "I think he felt his boss was not being fair with him, and he lost his temper and said things to his boss that he never should have said. And I'm convinced that was one of the earlier symptoms of his mental illness."

As a result of this behaviour, Cameron lost his position in June of 1994. Through the long summer that followed, his father tried to give his twenty-eight-year-old son gentle encouragement, to help get him back on track.

"You could see his self-confidence was very low during that period," he says, his voice slowing as he remembers the pain his son was enduring at the time.

"I knew that when he went in for interviews, he was putting his worst foot forward. I got him some help from one of these industrial psychologists, but that didn't really work out too well, either."

In October, there was an episode Wilson describes as "a big blow-up." To protect Cameron, he won't give details, but he does say his son was very upset about a situation that "really seemed to eat away at him." Wilson, who already had affiliations with the Clarke Institute of Psychiatry through his charitable work, contacted the facility.

"He got some help from psychiatrists, social workers, psychologists," he explains. "We had a hard time trying to find one that he related to, and actually the person that he related to best was a social worker."

At this stage, the family was hopeful. Though Cameron wasn't thrilled about seeking help, he recognized that he needed a hand. Inklings, at least, of progress. Then came the phone call, in the middle of the night, in the middle of December. Michael Wilson picked up the receiver. His son told him to rush over to the apartment, that someone was outside, watching him.

Wilson raced to his car and started driving across town, toward the apartment his son shared with friends. He was on a major street at about 3 a.m. when something caught his eye.

"There he was, walking along in his slippers and pyjamas, in mid-December. I took him home, and we got him down to the Clarke

Institute right after that. He spent some time in the Clarke off and on from that point."

The initial diagnosis, Wilson recalls, was something known as schizophreniform disorder. It has schizophrenia-like qualities, including delusions, but develops within a shorter time frame. The doctors said it was only a provisional diagnosis, and it remained fuzzy.

"They weren't quite sure whether this was going to lead to schizophrenia. We never really got a firm diagnosis," says Wilson.

Cameron hated being in the hospital. Not the facility, but the idea of being in a *psychiatric* hospital. He was afraid his friends would judge him weak, faulty, crazy. And so, with the exception of his very closest pal, he told no one. He also instructed his family that they were not to tell anyone, not even his roommates. He continued this self-imposed silence into January, when he made a suicide attempt with some over-the-counter medications. His sister says the stigma of mental illness robbed Cameron of precious support.

"His friends used to call and ask us what was the matter," says Lara. "And Cameron didn't want anybody to know; it was 'none of their business.' And these were his best friends that he grew up with in Ottawa. And it was really tough to say to them, 'I can't tell you anything.'"

Following the attempt to end his life, Cameron briefly rallied. After moving home to live with his parents, he told his father and his mother, Margie, he was not going to let this thing, this illness, get the better of him – that he would beat it. It was that same competitive spirit that had served him so well in so many other endeavours. During this period, Cameron also opened up, frequently, with his mom.

"Margie was with him all the time, and they had a number of pretty deep discussions. So it wasn't just me, or just the kids. It was all of us, and she was very, very much involved."

But for every step forward, Cameron struggled. The idea of being in "the loony bin," as he once called it, wore heavily on him. And because the setback seemed so insurmountable, at least in his mind, it was difficult for the young man to focus on the future.

"One of the things he said to me," says Wilson, "was, 'Dad, promise me you won't tell anybody what's wrong with me, because I'll never get a job again. People will think that I'm a schiz.' He felt that he was doomed if anybody found out where he was. The stigma issue was very, very tough on him. He said, 'I'll never be able to do the things that you and Geoff are doing.' So he really saw the black side of life going forward, and that was the sad part about it, that he couldn't open up to his friends."

He confided in only one, his closest. The rest of the time, he shared with his parents, either at home or up at the family farm. There, he'd allow those closest to glimpse the burden he was carrying, to lessen the load.

"He talked, but it was because he couldn't get answers; the doctors weren't able to give him the answers to the questions. I think the most troublesome thing to him was that they couldn't get the right mix for the medication, and all he could see was that the medication wasn't working, and he never had the confidence that it would work," says Wilson.

And with every treatment that failed, Cameron became more despondent. His lack of physical energy troubled him, too, especially given his athletic past. Over time, with shifting diagnoses and seemingly endless waits for the meds to work, he began to feel truly hopeless. It seemed even worse when doctors proposed taking Cameron off medication and trying electroconvulsive therapy. He told his parents he was getting increasingly frustrated.

"The doctors had told him that he was going to have the ECT treatment, and I don't think he looked forward to that with any enthusiasm or optimism," says Wilson. "It was in that week between telling him they were going to take him off his current medication before he got onto the ECT that he took his life."

Unlike many who end their lives, Cameron had given no warning to his family following his initial attempt. There may have been a slight hint to one close friend – but certainly nothing explicit.

Several years prior to Cameron's death, Michael Wilson was looking for a new cause. He'd always placed an emphasis on non-profit public service and had worked for more than a decade on behalf of the Canadian Cancer Society.

But that organization, Wilson knew, now had scores of thousands of employees and volunteers. It also was very prominent in the public mindset. Perhaps there was another cause, one that needed a boost in profile.

"So I decided I would work on behalf of mental illness. I didn't realize the irony of that," he says, "[with] what was going to happen a couple of years later."

It is a sad truth that Cameron's illness, in conjunction with the stigma associated with mental disorder, robbed him of support. He believed no one cared, that no one could understand. Yet his funeral was packed with friends, good people who cared about him and who told the family they would have been there for Cameron. Some even told Wilson that they themselves had suffered from mental illness and would have understood.

"When he died, there were a ton of young people at his funeral. They came from Ottawa, Montreal, and other places outside of Toronto as well. So he had lots of friends," says Wilson.

Friends who cared. And a family that still does. Which is why they agreed to speak.

"I would hope that people would take steps to seek help earlier," says Geoff. Like his father, he also expresses the wish that general practitioners could be a little more cautious about watching for symptoms of mental disorder and relaying them in a sensitive way to patients.

Lara, meanwhile, hopes Cameron's story chips away at the stigma, the stereotypes, the ignorance.

"It gets very frustrating when you hear people talking about 'that loony over there,' talking about someone who's not very stable. And they don't wonder *why* they're not stable," she says. "There are a lot of people in the world today that are crying out for some kind of attention. It could be your next-door neighbour, it could be the person you sit next to at work, it could be anyone. There's no way you can know just by looking at someone."

"A lesson from Cameron is that people should be talking to people about it," she continues. "If they confide in someone, that person should help by seeking support for them. If you know someone who is sick, call and see how you can get help."

When asked what he remembers most about his son, Michael Wilson stops to think for a minute. Then he smiles.

"Well, I think the thing that keeps coming back with Cameron is he had a great big laugh, and when he'd be on the phone with a friend, or downstairs having a beer with some buddies, then this great big laugh . . .

"That's the thing that keeps coming back."

As he savours the memory, Michael Wilson's piercing eyes seem to gaze inwards, to reflect. And in that flickering instant, they reveal incredible loss, and incredible love.

PAST LIVES

Diagnosing people posthumously is a decidedly risky business, especially when it comes to mental disorder. Virtually none of the diagnoses used by modern-day psychiatrists existed when Abraham Lincoln or Vincent van Gogh were alive. Researchers have pored over letters, journal entries, and other writings to try to gauge how these famous souls would have been diagnosed in the modern age. But even these reference materials can be questionable, because each reflects a mere moment in time — moments that may or may not have included exaggeration, understatement, or anything in between.

Here, we let you judge for yourself.

VIRGINIA WOOLF

"I believe these illnesses are in my case — how shall I express it? — partly mystical. Something happens in my mind. It refuses to go on registering impressions. It shuts itself up. It becomes chrysalis. I lie quite torpid, often with acute physical pain — as last year; only discomfort this. Then suddenly something springs."

— diary entry, September 10, 1929

F. SCOTT FITZGERALD

"I began to realize that for two years my life had been drawing on resources that I did not possess, that I had been mortgaging myself physically and spiritually up to the hilt. . . . I realized that in those two years, in order to preserve something — an inner hush, maybe, maybe not — I had weaned myself from all the things I used to love — that every act of life from the morning toothbrush to the friend at dinner had become an effort. I saw that for a long time I had not liked people and things, but only followed the rickety old pretense of liking."
— F. Scott Fitzgerald, "The Crack-Up," 1936

ABRAHAM LINCOLN

"I am now the most miserable man living. If what I feel were equally distributed to the whole human family, there would be not one cheerful face on earth. Whether I shall ever be better, I cannot tell. I awfully forebode I shall not. To remain as I am is impossible. I must die or be better it appears to me."
— letter to his law partner, January, 1841

EDGAR ALLAN POE

"My feelings at this moment are pitiable indeed. I am suffering under a depression of spirits such as I have never felt before. I have struggled in vain against the influence of this melancholy . . . I am wretched, and know not why. Console me — for you can. But let it be quickly — or it will too late. Write me immediately. Convince me that it is worth one's while — that it is at all necessary to live, and you will prove yourself indeed my friend."
— letter to a friend, September 11, 1835

LORD BYRON

"I am so bilious — that I nearly lose my head — and so nervous that I cry for nothing — at least today I burst into tears all alone by myself over a cistern of Gold fishes — which are not pathetic animals. . . . I have been excited — and agitated and exhausted mentally and bodily all this summer — till I really sometimes begin to think not only "that I shall die at top first" — but that the moment is not very remote. — I have had no particular cause of grief — except the usual accompaniments of all unlawful passions."
— letter to a friend, August, 1819

LEO TOLSTOY

"It is now clear to me that there was no difference between ourselves [the intellectuals of the day] and people living in a madhouse; at the time I only vaguely suspected this, and, like all madmen, I thought everyone except myself was mad."

— Leo Tolstoy, *Confession*, 1884

ROBERT SCHUMANN

"I was seized with the worst fear a man can have, the worst punishment Heaven can inflict — the fear of losing one's reason. It took so strong a hold of me that consolation and prayer, defiance and derision, were equally powerless to subdue it. . . . Ah, Clara! no one knows the suffering, the sickness, the despair, except those so crushed."

— letter to his wife, Clara, 1838

VINCENT VAN GOGH

"Well, well, after all, there are so many painters who are cracked in one way or another that little by little I shall be reconciled to it."

— letter to his brother, Theo, February 22, 1889

ROBERT BURNS

"The weakness of my nerves has so debilitated my mind that I dare not either review past events, or look forward into futurity; for the least anxiety, or perturbation in my breast, produces most unhappy effects on my whole frame. . . . I am quite transported at the thought that ere long, perhaps very soon, I shall bid an eternal adieu to all the pains, & uneasiness & disquietudes of this weary life; for I assure you I am heartily tired of it, and, if I do not very much deceive myself, I could contentedly & gladly resign it."

— letter to his family, December 27, 1781

SIR ISAAC NEWTON

"I am extremely troubled at the embroilment I am in, and have neither ate nor slept well this 12 month, nor have my former consistency of mind. . . . [I] am now sensible that I must withdraw from your acquaintance, and see neither you nor the rest of my friends any more, if I may but leave them quietly."

— letter to writer Samuel Pepys, 1693

KATHERINE BEST*
Health Care Administrator

Katherine Best has a few reasons to be nervous. These last five years off work, living on long-term disability, she's spent a lot of time at home. Her front door – one of several identical doors on this well-kept suburban street – bears a friendly *Welcome* sign, but Katherine is unaccustomed to visitors. And she's especially unaccustomed to talking about what's kept her here inside while her friends and neighbours – the rest of the world, it seems – are out working. "I've never talked about it with anybody in detail, other than my physician," she says softly. "Not even my friends or family."

Katherine is a compact, middle-aged woman with a round face, short brown hair, and three small earrings (two in her left ear). Dressed neatly in blue jeans and a tucked-in T-shirt with a maple leaf logo, she gives no clue she has anything an insurance company would classify as a disability. And yet as she starts to tell her story, the pain in her face is unmistakeable. At times, the tears spill over – silent tears, and she talks right through them, squeezing her eyes tight as if willing them away. "I've been the type who's kept everything on an intellectual level and has not explored emotion," she explains, and there is pain too in her quiet voice, in the steady slowness of these few words.

"My story is simple to tell," she says, "forty-seven years of madness and five years of stability."

Katherine Best's forty-seven years of madness began in an abusive home and began to end while working as a health care administrator, setting up a new emergency services system for Nova Scotia.

She'd gone into health care – first as a nurse, then as a nursing teacher, and eventually a senior executive in charge of emergency services for a one-thousand-bed hospital – because she wanted the kind of stability she'd never had growing up. "I grew up really poor in a dysfunctional and abusive family," she says. Her father was a fireman,

---

* The name Katherine Best is a pseudonym.

supporting six children – and a hefty alcohol bill – on one salary. Home then was city housing, a converted military barracks with plenty of cockroaches but just three rooms, and a shower shared with other families. Katherine and her sisters slept in one bed. And that was the least of their troubles.

"He was a really abusive man, my father. I think his idea of having kids was that he had a little pack of slaves that were to do his bidding. And whenever he said 'Jump,' you just said, 'How high?'" The man was a severe alcoholic, and Katherine believes he also had undiagnosed bipolar disorder. Her mother suffered from depression. "My doctor says I was in a bad gene pool," Katherine says with grim humour. As the oldest girl, she did a lot of the caring for her younger siblings, as well as trying to protect her mother from her father's abuse.

Katherine remembers nights when her father would come home drunk and round everyone up for a "kangaroo court," going one by one around the table, calling his daughters sluts or whores and saying he wished they'd get pregnant and get out of his house. "He was always drunk. He'd come home and get you up, and he'd have a gun and he'd hold it in front of you. And you always thought you could die at any time. . . . It was a nightmare. You always lived in fear.

"So I got out of that and went into nursing, basically because I didn't have money and I needed to have an education, because I was not going to stay in that kind of a situation."

With hospital shift work, and living in nurses' residence, she made it through university and graduated in 1972, when jobs were plentiful. Now, finally, she was safe and financially secure. She also enjoyed the work. "As it happened, I really loved it. So it proved to be a really good move."

Over the next two decades, her career took off. She wound up managing a budget of several million dollars and a staff of about one hundred. She was responsible for such tasks as negotiating a deal to buy a fleet of 150 new ambulances for the province.

Her bank account flourished in turn. The girl who had once worn hand-me-downs and survived on a diet of milk and bread for days at a stretch was now an independent woman wearing business suits, travelling back and forth, with a briefcase in hand, between her large office and expensive home.

It must have looked to all the world like a happy and successful life. She had, after all, achieved the North American dream, pulling herself out of dire circumstances through her own hard work, skill, and planning. She had traded in her old life for a new and infinitely better one. Except that, try as she might to outrun it, the old life stayed with her.

From the start, there was terrible guilt about leaving her siblings and mother, about "being free while others still lived there." And there was this chronic inability to enjoy her hard-won freedoms. "You live with fear and insecurity, [but then] when you leave it, somehow it's worse than when you were there. Which is surprising. I think you're used to living at such a high stress level that when the stress is gone, you don't really know how to live."

While in nursing school, Katherine became clinically depressed. She started seeing a psychiatrist, but that didn't help. "He did nothing for me, and over the years it just got worse and worse. After that I never wanted to see a doctor or talk about it to a doctor, because I thought they were all full of shit, basically." As her career became more successful, her inner world became ever more bleak, filled with a despair and anger she could not comprehend. To make the two worlds meet, she became "a great actress," hiding not only her misery but also her sexuality. "Another closet I lived in was the fact that I was gay, a closet I lived in until I was thirty-nine. So I lived in the closet about my father and what was going on at home. I lived in the closet about being gay. My relationships were with people in authority over me . . . and they were really closeted relationships."

For years, the acting worked; no one knew her secrets. But inside, she was no happier, and maintaining the facade only became more difficult with time. It was like living inside a balloon, watching the rubber stretch ever thinner, waiting for the big explosion. She would spend twelve hours at the office holding everything in and then let all the air out when she finally got home. "I could control it outside, because you have to. But at home it was awful. I had a little dog at the time, who I loved dearly, and I know I scared this poor little animal all the time. I just couldn't help it. . . . I'd bang the wall with my fists, I'd yell and I'd screech, and I knew I had to stop because the neighbours would hear. But it was so hard being outside and just keeping a lid on that all the time." Hard, too, to imagine this soft-spoken woman habitually pounding her fists on the walls.

Eventually, her irritability started leaking into the workplace. She became argumentative in business meetings, would snap at her secretary and even her boss. Her friends started noticing something was wrong. She was living with a woman, and that relationship started suffering, too. For all these reasons, she started believing that she must be like her father – an evil person. And always, her mind was racing. "I'd go to bed at night – boom, boom, boom with this and that. . . . I could never put my head to rest. Never."

The final break came one fateful Friday afternoon in 1996 when she walked out of her office furious over a series of disagreements with her colleagues. "My internal volcano exploded," she explains. "In a fugue state, I got up from my desk, put on my coat, picked up my briefcase, and walked out. . . . And that was it. I never went back."

Her family doctor referred her to a psychiatrist who prescribed an antidepressant and predicted she'd be back at work in a couple of weeks. Far from it. Three months later, she attempted suicide, swallowing prescription pills – "by then I had a truckload of pills that I was taking" – before making a desperate call to her psychiatrist. "I thought, Oh my God, I don't want to die. I just want the pain to stop."

She spent the next two months in a psychiatric hospital. Having worked in health care for twenty-five years, she now saw for the first time what life was like on the other side. And it shocked her. "I didn't know what to expect, but as a patient, oh my Lord, you're totally depersonalized. You're not a person, you're a patient, and all the patients are basically treated the same. . . . They just put me on medication. They never saw my behaviour or talked to me. But they would continue to increase dosages or change the medications."

Echoing many people who've spent time in psychiatric facilities, she says she has fond memories of some of her fellow patients. "Some of the nicest people in there were the patients, because at least you could talk to them. At least you felt human with them." One kind man who'd been a patient for years acted as her guardian, showing her how the system worked. "I wouldn't have known how to survive. Ernest took me under his wing because he was seasoned." And there were plenty of "seasoned" patients who, she says, "sat there and sat there for months and months. It reminded me of the old asylum days when . . . you could stay there forever."

At forty-seven, in a psychiatric hospital for the first time in her life, Katherine Best finally was diagnosed with rapid-cycling bipolar disorder – mania causing the racing mind, depression causing the deep despair and self-loathing. She thought her diagnosis was all just "melodrama or something. I guess I didn't see it as real." The drugs she was given left her increasingly incapacitated; she says she lost her memory, her powers of concentration, her ability to read or drive a car. "I was like a zombie." But it wasn't all bad. For the first time in a very long while, her mind fell quiet. "You couldn't bring up thoughts if you wanted to. It was like a blank, and that was such a relief, a rest."

A concerned friend and her sister, both of whom worked in health care, pushed for her discharge. She believes this is why she was released sooner than many of the other patients. "Unless somebody knows you and acts as your ombudsman, you could be in there forever. Because once you've been on the drugs, your memory goes, you can't concentrate, you don't think about anything."

Katherine is not anti-medication; she takes mood-stabilizing drugs to this day. But her diagnosis can be tricky to treat; it took almost two years before her psychiatrist found the right combination of meds. This was a new psychiatrist (assigned to her after her hospitalization), the person she credits with giving her a new life. "I had such disregard for psychiatry and psychiatrists. But right from the start she was phenomenal. . . . She's a fantastic listener. She keeps giving you hope. . . . And there has not been one thing she's ever told me that hasn't proven to be the case. I trust her implicitly."

It was the psychotherapy – begun once the meds had been sorted out – that she says wrought the most significant changes. With her therapist, she started making connections, understanding why she behaved as she had. "She took me from dealing with everything at an intellectual level to an emotional level. I was forty-seven, and I had never allowed myself, ever, to get into that stuff. In fact, I just totally blocked it. I didn't know what stability was, emotionally. And I could not believe there would be a light at the end of the tunnel. And she kept encouraging me, [saying] 'Give it time, it takes work.' And I started to believe that there was something that could be done."

Her biggest issue has been work; for all those years it had defined her, and then it was gone. "I tried so hard to get back into the workplace. Because of my past, security was everything to me. I worked to get to a place where I had my best earning years to prepare for retirement. That was gone. I went on a pension which, of course, isn't near to what my salary was, and doesn't grow, and doesn't allow me to save money or to have any real earning power." Since her hospitalization, she's had only one job, which lasted eight months and was arranged so that she could keep her disability benefits. It was a long way from what she'd done as a senior manager. "I got a job at the museum, packing boxes and materials that got sent out to schools," she says with a level voice. "But it was really good, because it was part-time, limited-to-no-stress."

Last fall, the position was terminated, and she hasn't worked since. Over the years, she's felt worse about her unemployment than about her mental illness. "I didn't mind telling people that I'd had an illness and that it was a mental health problem. It was harder for me to answer the question 'What are you doing now?' That was the thing I was lying about. You go from being a fairly high-profile, high-paid person to being nobody, because when people meet you, one of the first things they ask is, 'What do you do?'"

Today, she feels fortunate that her salary was high enough to provide for disability payments that keep her "comfortable." Mindful of her finances, she sold the large house and moved into a townhouse. Her new abode has the bright, polished look of a designer home, decorated with shiny hardwood floors, modern furniture, and primary colours. She's invested much time in making it hers. And yet she knows that her future lies beyond the confines of home, no matter how comfortable it may be. "I know I'll never be able to go back to what I did. I don't have the ability to handle that kind of stress. [But] I need to be with people more. So if I had a job part-time, with minimal stress and with people, that would be fine. And I don't care what it is I do."

For a moment, she allows herself to picture the possibilities. Gardening, for example, has always been a love of hers – she's good with her hands and built her own garden in her previous home, complete with hot tub, rock garden, and pond. "I drive by one of the local nurseries up the street and they're looking for people to work, and I'd just love to walk in and say, 'Here I am, and I'm available!' Something like that would be ideal."

But working even part-time would mean losing her disability cheques, her main source of financial security. So for the time being, her life remains in limbo. "I really need to volunteer," she says anxiously. "I have to force myself to get out of the house. And I know the longer I don't do that, then the harder it will be."

Five years after she entered the psychiatric hospital, Katherine Best is still finding her place, and that is scary and exciting all at once. Painful as this whole experience has been, she looks back on it now and feels grateful for the chance to start over. "I would have lived my life being absolutely painfully miserable. I never would have gotten past that without being sick. So it's a blessing to know that, knock on wood, if things continue to work, this is going to be my life. I don't ever have to go back into that painful, painful thing. Yes, getting sick was the best thing that ever happened to me, really and truly."

What she hopes others will learn from her experience is that the fine line that separates madness from sanity is scarcely a line at all. She knows; she's seen both sides. "Anybody can cross that line," she says. "And you *never* think it's going to happen to you."

She apologizes for talking too much, explaining how rare it still is for her to speak with people at length. She looks genuinely concerned. As she stands in the doorway, waving goodbye, she is smiling, but her sadness, her solitude, is plain to see. She's better than she was, but she's not quite there yet. Her search for a new future – a full life to replace the old, troubled one – continues.

EDMOND YU
Student

On February 20, 2002, it rained in Toronto. It seems to rain or snow every year on the anniversary of Edmond Yu's death. That's not to suggest the weather somehow is sympathetic; it just has a habit of being grey on this particular day.

Each year since his death in 1997, a group of people gathers at noon in a small park in downtown Toronto. They come to this place because, for a brief period during Edmond's life, he lived here. It was a place where, despite his homelessness and suffering, Edmond Yu found a measure of solace and safety. A home where, despite his cascading thoughts, he could simply *be*. Edmond slept on the concrete outside a public washroom, where the overhang of the roof offered some protection from the elements. People continue to choose the location for the same reason (along with its proximity to toilets and hot running water). On this day, nearly a dozen sleeping bags have been left unzipped to air out until their owners return. The frigid air is so moist the bags will be damp for several nights to come.

The memorial, as always, is simple: a few speakers, a couple of songs, fragments of memories. Some of those who address the small crowd are activists who believe Edmond is symbolic of wider problems – the lack of safe housing for psychiatric survivors, the need for better police training, the paucity of compassion and tolerance in a country as wealthy and diverse as Canada. So numerous are the related issues that there's the occasional awkward moment when it feels like Edmond has become a multi-purpose poster boy. Very few of those attending actually knew him – either as friends, fellow survivors, or as mental health workers. Those who did, recall an extraordinary and complex man.

"I remember Edmond's face . . ." says Raymond Cheng, who met him at a program he runs for people from Southeast Asia with mental health issues. "There's a look in someone's eyes when you see great wisdom. But I also saw the great and profound sadness of someone who knew he was never really going to fit in."

As a young boy growing up in Hong Kong, Edmond Wai-Hong Yu did more than fit in. Whether it was in academics or athletics, the schoolbooks or the schoolyard, Edmond always pushed himself to excel. In addition to acing his studies, he shone at a number of sports, including kung fu, badminton, basketball, and boxing. (He won a city boxing championship in his early teens – and was a whiz at chess.)

"When he had his mind set on something," says his sister Katherine, "nothing could stand in his way. He would really go for it."

Despite that drive, Edmond also had a softer side. He was devoted to his family. As a teenager, he'd pick up small gifts for his two sisters, delighting in their pleasure. When Edmond's older brother left home, his father became his sole male role model. The two were exceptionally close.

In Edmond's mid-teens, however, Mr. Yu became seriously ill. The local clinic shared neither the diagnosis (liver cancer) nor the prognosis (poor) with the family, instead administering an expensive treatment regime that did little to improve the condition. When Edmond learned the truth after his father died in 1981, he was outraged. The clinic had betrayed them. "This was quite a turmoil for Edmond; he was closest to my father," recalls Katherine.

So searing was the experience that it strengthened Edmond's determination to become a doctor, a healer. In 1982, he brought that dream to Canada when he and his mother immigrated, joining Edmond's older brother. Accepted at York University, he spent two years in premed. And, just as in Hong Kong, he shone.

"He was brilliant, absolutely brilliant," says former classmate Dr. David Persaud. "He was the top science student in the entire university. Only four of us got into medical school that year." Edmond was one of them, earning a scholarship to the University of Toronto. In the fall of 1984, Edmond Yu walked into the historic lecture halls and began the hard work of becoming a doctor.

It was no surprise when he achieved outstanding marks in his first term. But things changed the following semester. Subtly, Edmond withdrew. He started studying from home, avoiding campus except when exams or group projects required him to be there. When he had to do clinical work in hospital settings, other med students noticed that Edmond wasn't his usual caring self. "He seemed to have difficulty interacting with patients in stressful circumstances," recalls Dr. Persaud. "When you're a medical student, you're often thrown into a situation where you have to see a patient with terminal AIDS or terminal cancer, and there may be a family member there. Circumstances like that are very, very stressful. And I heard a few rumours that he had difficulty coping with that."

The initial signs that not all was well were detected an ocean away by Katherine, who was then living in Hong Kong. Her elder brother and mother made increasingly worried calls to her, saying Edmond's behaviour was changing. He was convinced there were unusual smells permeating the family's home and accused his brother of spraying poisons. At one point it escalated into an argument so serious that Edmond was asked to move out.

Edmond called, too, talking in an increasingly disjointed fashion about conspiracies and plots against him. The young man who had always been so meticulous and rational was plagued with thoughts that simply did not make sense. "He started to talk about things that were not normal," she recalls. "I realized at that point there was something wrong with him."

Katherine flew to Canada to find a situation more serious than she had imagined. The university said Edmond had been making obscene phone calls to some of his classmates. He was also sporadically following a woman he had a crush on, sometimes sitting outside her house. She'd phone the Yu family, frightened, and they would come pick Edmond up. Over and over.

His paranoia was also growing. On one visit to his apartment, Katherine saw dramatic evidence he was becoming more unwell. "He said the people in his building, as well as in nearby buildings, were spies," she says. "He believed there were satellites planted in his building – even in his own apartment – watching him." He also insisted there was nothing unusual about these beliefs and refused to see a doctor.

For those who loved Edmond, the options began to narrow. The family considered obtaining an order for psychiatric examination. But for a judge to grant that order, the family would have to prove either that Edmond had threatened or attempted to hurt himself or someone else, or that he was unable to care for himself. Though unwell, Edmond was not that far gone. And so, Katherine reluctantly took matters into her own hands. She visited Edmond again, pushing relentlessly for him to be assessed. He asked her to leave, but she continued to challenge him.

"And then he slapped me in the face."

It was totally out of character for Edmond, but his action did meet the legal criteria to have him taken to hospital for examination. Six police officers handcuffed him and took him to a psychiatric hospital, where he was forcibly injected with the antipsychotic haloperidol (Haldol). His medical records indicate psychosis was present, and his break from reality "may have been precipitated by the stress of medical school and a possible failed romantic relationship."

Medicated, Edmond was soon allowed to take day passes from the hospital. Katherine recalls meeting him for one of them. "He wanted to go to U of T, and the first place he went was into the medical school, the lecture halls. Even after all these years, it still really moves me. He just walked around the lecture hall, touched the chairs, touched the tables, everything. I knew it really hurt."

So did the treatment. Some people experience extreme side-effects with certain psychotropic drugs – and Edmond Yu was one of them. "When he was on medication," says Katherine, "he seemed to be a totally different person. All he could do was eat and sleep. He was completely non-communicative. His hands were so shaky, he couldn't even hold a bowl of soup properly. The soup would always spill. He couldn't even control going to the toilet. He was such an energetic person, and then suddenly it seemed he could not control anything."

Edmond was suffering extreme side-effects, consisting of involuntary spasms and tremors and tics. Unknown at the time was that people of Asian descent can be particularly sensitive to antipsychotic drugs. The agony Edmond endured would forever taint his view of psychiatric medications.

Med school this year would be out of the question, because of the side-effects, and because he'd missed the first month of classes. He stopped taking his medication and planned to return to university the following year. But since he would not adhere to the drugs, a psychiatrist refused to issue a letter stating Edmond was fit to attend classes.

"After he was refused," says Katherine, "he knew his dream was over."

More turmoil was to strike the Yu family when Edmond's older brother was diagnosed with terminal cancer. Edmond, who had briefly been back on medication, stopped taking it the day after the funeral in early 1987. Then his illness spiralled. Overtaken by paranoia and suspicion, he feared those closest to him were conspiring to harm him. He talked non-stop about his special influence over world affairs. On occasion, he was verbally abusive. Perhaps most troubling, he began burning some of his most personal belongings. Photographs, books, clothes. He simply took them out onto the driveway and set them on fire.

"It's sort of like he wanted to get rid of his past," says Katherine. "He just wanted to burn it, tear it down, to have nothing of that past."

Despite the crushing disappointment of losing his planned career, Edmond eventually sought other work. He applied for a series of low-paying jobs: salon hair-washer, security guard, mover, fish-scaler. Sometimes the jobs lasted a few days, sometimes just one. Edmond was trying to find a place for himself. "One thing I really admired in him," says Katherine, "is in spite of all the broken dreams and heartache, he never gave up striving. Even though these were jobs he would never have considered in the past."

But her admiration was tinged with frustration. Having Edmond at home was difficult. In the end, the family gave him a choice: take the medications or leave. In the summer of 1988, he left.

Edmond began to drift. From housing, to hostels – where he complained of being beaten and robbed – to the street. He made the odd trip home, usually a monthly visit to pick up his welfare cheque. His clothes were becoming ragged, he carried a single bag of dried food. In December 1988, the family found him living outside the public washroom in a downtown park. Concerned that he was unable to care for himself, they applied for another order for examination. It was granted. Edmond spent more than three months in hospital, much of it making successful legal challenges against plans to medicate him.

Over the next few years, a kind of pattern set in. On three occasions between 1989 and 1992, Edmond struck or pushed strangers and was charged with assault. The Yu family pleaded with judges to send Edmond to hospital instead of jail, for treatment instead of incarceration. During his last stay in custody, Edmond did receive medication. Unfortunately, he developed unusual and almost intolerable side-effects.

"After he was released," says Katherine, "he was so sick, getting sicker and sicker. He came home, he couldn't eat, he couldn't drink, he couldn't move. He was shaking involuntarily, consistently." Edmond was in such terrible shape that he was receptive to offers of help from his family. Katherine rushed him to an emergency ward; he agreed to remain in hospital for treatment and stayed for two months.

Upon release, a social worker found him a room at a boarding home for people with psychiatric illnesses. A house rule stipulated that all tenants must agree to remain on their medication. Edmond initially refused. Katherine says she was so desperate that she threatened to sever all ties with her brother if he did not consent. He relented and signed an agreement to adhere to the prescribed medication. But much of his time at Rainbow House, from mid-1992 to April 1996, was spent in bed. A combination of the meds and inactivity led to a dramatic weight gain. Katherine encouraged him to exercise, get out walking, visit the library.

And then, toward the end of his stay at the boarding house, Edmond began to rediscover simple pleasures. "There was a sense of wonder," says Katherine. "When we took him to Niagara Falls, or to Centre Island, he seemed to be like a child. He'd laugh, watch the fireworks, and really enjoy life." Edmond also started showing concern for others close to him, once again doing favours for his mother and sisters. "That was the time," she says, "when I knew I was interacting with a person. A person who has a heart."

Edmond, for the last time, had stopped his medication. Katherine believes he was at a stage where enough remained in his system to keep him stable – without the side effects. And, after all he'd been through, she can sympathize with his attempt to do without the drugs. "He might have wanted to give it a try," she concedes. "After all those years, he wanted to give it a try." He also decided to move out, to find some measure of independence. He rented an apartment in a building that houses many people with psychiatric backgrounds.

Outreach worker Bob Rose says it's not unusual for long-term boarding-home residents to make such decisions. "They're taking their medication, they're in treatment," he says, "and life is very empty. And they get up and leave. And the first thing they say is: 'I'm going to stop taking the medication. I'm going to rent an apartment. I'm going to live my life.' It's quite common for people, in that early period, to do that quite successfully, to be energized, to feel more human, to feel like themselves."

Edmond also started to frequent a local drop-in for people who call themselves "psychiatric survivors," meaning they've survived the mental health system. Then–program co-ordinator Louis Dionne recalls their conversations being extraordinary. "He had this philosophical bent. He was always after this point of equilibrium between the possible and the impossible, between the visible and the invisible, between life and death. So he was fascinating."

He was also eager to be around other people. "He liked being engaged," says Dionne. "In fact, I think that's what he craved. He really wanted conversation and presence and contact."

That fall, Edmond Yu was evicted after a dispute with the landlord. He'd apparently been making noise, singing and banging in his room at odd hours. He left with little more than the multiple layers of clothes on his back. That's when Bob Rose, who works at that neighbourhood drop-in, first saw Edmond. It was a late November day, and Edmond was standing outside the rooming house with a cheque in his hand. "And he was all layered up," says Rose. "The stuff was all new, all black. He was quite a distinguished looking man." Edmond wore a total of twelve layers on his upper body: eight sweaters, two down-filled vests, two parkas.

Rose, who detected something "exceptional" about him, would spend the next month trying to establish some sort of trust. Edmond had become a resourceful nomad, wandering to the Scott Mission for meals, to church basements for shelter, to the library, the park, Chinatown. He was in no rush to seek either housing or treatment, nor was Rose going to push him. "This is a person who's had a complicated history in terms of homelessness and mental health. And this is a person you have to be careful with, because he will run. If you do this wrong, you're gonna be just like everybody else who ever met him. So we wanted to be careful not to fall into the same trap."

Rose and Dionne were not the only people on whom Edmond left an impression. At the Scott Mission he made quite an impact. Employee Cristine Bonadonna says Edmond could not be overlooked: "He had a quick tongue, very funny, full of life and spunk. That stands out a lot with men who are very isolated, who keep to themselves, who don't want to talk. Here's this person that's, like, in your face." A co-worker described his smile as "just beautiful, it was just so infectious. The smile of an eight-year-old kid on a man's body."

One of Edmond Yu's many temporary homes was a small branch of the Toronto Public Library. He visited daily, spreading his belongings out on the bench beside him. Occasionally he would mend his clothing; over time he sewed an entire knapsack. His striking features and nomadic presence led employees to nickname him "Lawrence of Arabia." Librarian Andrea Yermy has a vivid mental image of Edmond: "There was a meditative way about him. His movements were very precise, slow almost, in a calculated way but not in a catatonic way like some of the people here. And he had the most wonderful laughter."

Another of Edmond's regular stops was the Tibet Shoppe, a store specializing in Buddhist books and materials. When lucid, he'd converse with owner Gelek Gyaltong on topics ranging from Tibetan independence to spirituality. He was fascinated by ritual and Tibetan religious artifacts. "When he was lucid, he was very intelligent," says Gyaltong. "He was very up on the Tibetan issue, very well up on the history of China. He had a vast general knowledge and could carry on a conversation really well."

During an open-stage party celebrating the winter solstice, Edmond got onstage at the drop-in – insulated by all his layers – and sang "Born Free." He also sang "Yesterday," and those who knew him could not help but be moved by the lyrics. At other times he meditated while standing on his head. Played a brilliant game of chess while strategizing aloud. Carried a Scott Mission worker around on his back, played the piano, sang hymns.

"He was not," says Bob Rose, "your ordinary madman."

But the reality was that the combination of winter, homelessness, and illness were beginning to wear Edmond Yu down. At the solstice party he allowed the drop-in workers to take a look at his feet. "They were extremely callused," says Rose. "They were not frostbitten, but they were homeless feet."

As the weather worsened through January, Edmond's laughter did not come as easily. But still he did not complain, nor did he speak of his own suffering, except to note that "reality is sometimes painful." Edmond's ability to detach from his own plight gave him the aura, say some, of a Buddhist monk. "I've encountered few people who are that able to rise above their own level of discomfort, of physical pain, and just disregard it. It was, to him, irrelevant," recalls Louis Dionne.

It was, however, clear that Edmond was deteriorating. He confided to Bob Rose that he grappled constantly with the painful question "What purpose do I have in this world?" It's a sentiment Rose says is not uncommon among people in Edmond's situation: "This sense that there is no purpose, that they have no purpose, that society doesn't make it easy for them to find that purpose. About all they have is illness. And poverty. And stigma."

Edmond eventually agreed that he would like to find housing. Rose took him to one potential home, where tenants who met with him found his non-stop talking objectionable. Other options were explored, but with Edmond in this condition, there weren't very many.

As the temperature dropped, the pair discussed the possibility of hospitalization and eventually agreed on checking Edmond into a non-medical "safe house" for people in crisis. A forced hospital stay, Rose feared, would destroy the tentative trust that had been established.

The first night there, Edmond did not remove a single item of his multi-layered clothing. The second day, he set a piece of paper on fire in the kitchen sink. Rose started to think about hospitalization. That evening, however, Edmond appeared calmer. He allowed someone working at the safe house to tend to his callused feet.

On the morning of February 20, 1997, Edmond got up early and made breakfast for everyone, including staff. He said he had appointments, then left for the day. Outside, it was grey and overcast. Late in the afternoon, he wound up at a bus stop at the bottom of a major Toronto thoroughfare. For reasons we will never truly know, Edmond struck a woman in the face, then boarded a bus. Authorities would later say he told them she had been following him for days, staring at him every time he turned around.

The driver ordered everyone off the bus and left Edmond alone with the doors locked. Three police officers, one of whom told his colleagues "a nutbar" was involved, got on the bus and tried to persuade Edmond to leave with them. At one point, say the police, things were going well; it looked like he would depart voluntarily and go to hospital. But then the situation turned. Edmond drew a hammer from his jacket and raised it.

"I watched while he waggled his right wrist with the hammer in it," says one witness who had a view from an adjacent streetcar. "Then the movement of his wrist stopped, and seconds passed, when I heard what I thought initially was a cap gun. I could see the red flash of the gun, and the body slumped."

Constable Lou Pasquino started firing. He would later testify that he feared for his life. The first bullet hit Edmond directly in the throat and smashed into his vertebrae. A traumatized witness said a look of sheer astonishment crossed Edmond's face, as if he could not believe what had just happened. The shots continued. A second entered the side of Edmond's head and passed through his spinal cord.

Edmond Wai-Hong Yu, born October 2, 1961, was spinning and falling and dying as the third bullet grazed the back of his skull. He collapsed to the floor.

The first paramedic on the scene could not feel a pulse, but a sensor picked up a faint heartbeat. He attempted to place a tube in Edmond's throat to get his lungs going again, but the damage from the bullet rendered the task impossible. Within minutes, Edmond – in the neutral shorthand of the paramedic – "flatlined."

Gelek Gyaltong, when he learned of Edmond's death, phoned his wife – who is also a devout Buddhist. She was in India, visiting the Dalai Lama. On the night of that phone call, on the other side of the world, the Tibetan spiritual leader lit candles for Edmond Yu.

Two months after Edmond's death, the unit that investigates shootings by police in Ontario cleared the officers of any wrongdoing. Its press release stated that "events unwound quickly and a tragedy occurred."

Two years later, the inquest into his death wrapped up. It had been, like Edmond's life, a complex affair. A total of forty-seven witnesses, many of whom had very different agendas and perspectives, took the stand.

The police explained how, in their judgement, Edmond's hammer posed a potentially lethal threat. Constable Pasquino said he fired in self-defence, fearing for his personal safety and the safety of his fellow officers.

A police trainer testified that the best scenario would have occurred if the officers had not even boarded the bus. He also suggested they might have been too close to Edmond. "The number-one cardinal rule is: Move slowly and never invade their personal space," he said. If not, "You may be confirming the paranoia in the mind of the person you're dealing with. If you do that, the chances of escalation are greater."

Outreach workers decried the lack of safe and affordable housing. Specifically, they pointed out the virtual absence of accommodations that will tolerate the unusual behaviours of someone with a serious mental disorder. It was also noted that treating mental disorder is not always as simple as taking a pill.

"We like to approach mental illness like surgery: You cut the person open, you sew them back up, you send them out like nothing's happened. Well, it's not like that. The medication people take dampens things. For some people it resolves it completely, for others it just dampens it – it doesn't make it go away," says Rose.

Recommendations from the inquest included better police training, more "safe houses," and more research into non-medical forms of treatment for schizophrenia. But the jury also acknowledged that there were times when Edmond lashed out, and urged that it be made easier to hospitalize someone who poses a threat to public safety.

"Hopefully, with all of these recommendations, we will prevent similar deaths," said Katherine at the time. "I just want to look forward, instead of backward."

There are other Edmond Yus across Canada. Homeless, non-compliant, non-trusting. How best to deal with them? Hospital? Jail? Supportive housing? Forced medication? More safe houses?

There is, in all these questions, a common thread: Is there a place for the Edmond Yus of this world? And does society deem it a priority to help them find it?

"Edmond was a sick person," says Katherine. "But his sickness shouldn't make him less than human."

On the first anniversary of Edmond's death, Bob Rose made an impassioned address to the crowd attending his memorial. He wore a black vest, much like those Edmond had favoured. He held a hammer up before the crowd. "Edmond died with a hammer in his hand . . . much smaller than this hammer. And you know, I've always seen this tool to be a beautiful creation. It's used to make things, to build things. . . .

"Last night, someone – a stranger unknown to me – left this hammer on my desk. And they left a note beside it. And the note said, 'Build homes, build homes, build homes.' So I think, yes, Edmond's spirit is very close to us today."

A different version of this story first appeared in the Toronto Star *in October 1998. With Katherine's blessing, it helped raise nearly*

$20,000, money that was the genesis for a housing initiative in Edmond's name. The non-profit goal, which has a wide range of community support, is to operate transitional housing for high-need homeless psychiatric survivors in Toronto. It's called the Edmond Yu Safe House Project.

Donations can be made to Parkdale Activity-Recreation Centre, 1499 Queen Street West, Toronto, ON M6R 1A3. Please indicate in the memo line of your cheque that the donation is for the Edmond Yu Safe House. Income tax receipts will be issued for donations exceeding ten dollars.

CHAPTER 2 WHAT IT FEELS LIKE

—*m*—

Unless you've been there, it can be pretty difficult to imagine what it's like to suffer from a mental disorder. What does it truly *feel* like to experience the delusions or voices that come with schizophrenia? To soar with the unbridled euphoria of a mania? To shake with the heart-numbing fear of a panic attack?

Short of actually having the disorder, there are very few ways of comprehending what it's like to be inside someone else's head. We could rattle off lists of clinical symptoms, but that would get dull pretty fast. It also wouldn't really give you a visceral sense of the experience.

Yet all of us are curious. Scientists, in fact, have tried to give other folks a taste of what mental disorder feels like. One of the most intriguing efforts is a virtual-reality setup which, using specially enhanced audio and visual effects, attempts to transport the subject into the mind of someone with schizophrenia. You actually hear those internal voices in a manner that those with the disorder say comes close to their reality.

Since we couldn't package that simulator with this book, we figured we'd opt for something just as compelling: We asked people to write, in their own words, what it felt like for *them*.

Selecting the stories you are about to read was a difficult task. So difficult, there were moments when we ourselves struggled with feelings akin to anxiety and panic – and we're really not kidding. (Don't be surprised if there's a sequel to this book; there's still plenty of great material!)

In the end, we settled on these eight narratives, because of their raw descriptive power and because of the range of experiences they represent. What we were surprised to discover, at the end, was that all of them were written by women. It wasn't planned, there's no conspiracy – it just happened. (Interesting, though, that we did receive far more submissions from women than from men – perhaps an indication that women are still more willing to open up about their innermost thoughts and feelings.)

The eight women you're about to meet have all been there, done that, *felt* that.

ANDREA WOODSIDE
On Bipolar Disorder

Some sources will tell you that manic depression, or bipolar disorder, as it's also known, rarely shows itself much before the age of eighteen. But ask any of my friends, teachers, or family – any of those brave souls who travelled with me through my childhood – and they will vigorously dispute that claim.

My constant companion for as long as I can remember has been this illness. I remember asking my father when I was six years old if jumping off the roof of our house would kill me; the pain I felt had become so unbearable that I could not contemplate anything as remote as my seventh birthday. I can't recall his (surely horrified) reaction; I only remember feeling confident that I had an out.

For me, a rapid cycler, mood changes are like gunfire in the trenches – bang, bang, bang. Light, dark, light, dark. I don't know if it's possible to switch a light on and off as quickly as my brain manages to switch between euphoria and devastation.

I have spent most of my life feeling as though I will never join the human race. It's as though I live in a cage where I can hear the world but it cannot hear me. Now, in my thirties, I see this simply as a manifestation of my illness, which has a way of making the ordinary seem threatening and frightening. Paranoia is more than an occasional visitor. I have sat on the subway, convinced that others were laughing at me; I have left parties after an hour, certain that the guests thought I had no right to be among them. Manic depression can make that girl in *The Exorcist* (at her writhing, screaming, priest-hating worst) look like someone you would ask to babysit your three-year-old. But I own my illness. And it will be part of me for the rest of my life. I can't turn my back on it.

I have been asked if I see my illness as a tragedy, or at least as something that's robbed me of anything of vital importance. Sometimes I do. I think back on what it has prevented me from doing. I never finished high school, nor attended university – something I am still self-conscious about. But stress is a killer; it can initiate the descent into depression, the rise into mania. I have learned to be vigilant about avoiding those situations that will exacerbate my disease.

The illness also destroys relationships, chewing them up, spitting them out. I mourn the friendships I have lost. My behaviour – especially when manic – has alienated friends and lovers. In some cases, I have never been able to reconnect with them.

And yet, I can't say that I think of myself as tragically touched. It is like being born with red hair or brown, one eye or three; you know nothing different, so what does it matter? We all have a cross to bear. Mine just makes me crazy.

My dear friend Carol has likened my illness to diving off the dock at her cottage. When depressed, I enter a darkness I never thought could exist, a place with weeds so tall and tangled they threaten to pull me under. The sun can't penetrate the water's surface and I find myself disoriented. I swim, sputter, struggle, unsure if I'll surface or succumb.

And then, without warning, after hours, days, or weeks in these treacherous waters, I see land. The shore that was a mere speck across the waves when I first jumped off that dock is suddenly within reach. Among the pine trees, the moss-covered rocks and sweet-smelling sand, is the promise of safety, terra firma. I fall on the ground, thanking something up above for pulling me out just one more time. I don't for a moment imagine that I won't wind up underwater again; I just hope that it won't come too soon.

Of course, what goes down must eventually come up. Or so it is with this illness.

I wake up – maybe weeks, sometimes months later – hoping I haven't slept with someone I shouldn't have. I wonder if I'll get a Visa bill informing me that I am the owner of four new dishwashers and $1,800 worth of shoes. I tally up the countless and embarrassing hours spent drinking myself into erratic but necessary sleep, regaling my friends with endless stories – like the time I got stoned in a park with a complete stranger and had sex with him under the swings. All inhibitions, all sense of self-preservation, go out the window when I am manic.

The actor Patty Duke, a woman I respect very much, once bought a plane in Las Vegas while manic. I believe she bought it for a man she had met and married the day before. While I can't compete with that, I have some pretty interesting souvenirs myself, including a lovely martini shaker from Tiffany. (I have never had a martini in my life.) Incidentally, Tiffany's return policy leaves something to be desired.

The mania that comes after the crushing darkness is what I call the divine payback, and probably why manic depression hasn't killed me. The belief that the world is a truly beautiful place is what has kept me going long past my seventh birthday. And while I have done some remarkably stupid things while manic, I have also touched God, or at least the hem of his gown. It is the most extraordinary feeling, which I can only liken to having sight restored after a lifetime of blindness. I am renewed with the knowledge of every human being's staggering potential, of every joyous feeling that has existed since the beginning of time.

I feel awful for the unipolars. What do they do for fun?

I've been hospitalized a number of times and am a graduate of several Canadian and British psychiatric institutions. On various psych wards, I have heard inhuman screaming at all hours of the day and night. I have seen one particularly memorable "rehabilitation room" – in this case containing a dilapidated pool table, an old radio that didn't work, and a few dying plants – set on fire by a man who thought Satan lived in the utility closet. I have seen life-and-death struggles over the television remote control, and I have seen segregation. I was once tied to a bed for twenty-four hours in the hope that I might "co-operate." I was refusing to take a medication that came with the most remarkable side effects, namely instantaneous coma, as far as I could tell. Bra confiscated, iron bars on the windows, and not a bedsheet in sight. I have been in hospitals I could swear were jails.

Someone stands out in particular – a man I shall call George. He was about fifty, very tall, very thin, and dressed as if he'd just walked out of a Harrods fitting room. It turns out he was a stockbroker of some renown, and, like all good brokers, was deeply involved in a game of golf. For the first week of one of my hospitalizations, there came the *thunk*, *thunk* of his golf ball against the wall, at 1 a.m.,

3 a.m., 4 a.m., 6 a.m. Imagine his joy when he became convinced he'd won a qualifying PGA tournament.

George crashed a few days later, and when he did, he bore no resemblance to the man playing golf on Ward 5. For days, he lay on his bed, sweaty, naked, and dirty, often curled up in a fetal position as though he were dead. Occasionally, his screams shattered the ward's drug-enforced silence. No one rushed to his side.

After George recovered, he described his darkness to me. Imagine, he whispered, being cut up in little pieces then being thrown into a vat of acid, only you're still alive, and you're screaming for someone to help you, and no one can, and there's no ladder so you can't climb out, and then . . .

And then, George, you're back on terra firma. For a while.

How psychic pain can be that visceral, I do not know. I only know that George spoke the truth. And sometimes when you're in that vat of acid, you just have to breathe through it, like you're birthing something of magnificent proportions.

One thing this illness has not destroyed is my ambition. I have managed to rise to an upper-managerial level in the communications field. I have worked very hard to get to this point. But I worry about my employer finding out about my illness; close calls are scary. Recently, a colleague strolled into my office and happened to eye my bottle of valproic acid, which sat on my desk in anticipation of my noon dose. He picked it up, studied it, and announced that his best friend was bipolar and took valproic. Silence hung in the air. I coughed, looked at the floor, coughed again. I told him that it was for seizures.

Indeed, the drug has been used with some success for epileptic seizures, but I wondered if he bought it, and spent days avoiding him in the halls, at the coffee maker, by the photocopier. I am not ashamed of my illness; I simply cannot disclose in my workplace. I am afraid I could be fired. And if my clients find out, they might ask that I be removed from their business.

I don't feel like I lied. Manic depression is, in a way, like a seizure. It seizes you, spins you out of control, robs you of time – seconds, days, months – and then throws you back on the floor where it all started.

I believe that one day I will be able to tell people, if it comes up, that I have an illness, one no different than heart disease or diabetes. I was born this way, I live this way. It's okay.

I believe that, one day, my company drug plan will pay for my meds and I won't have to worry that someone at the insurance company will inform my boss that I have a mental illness; until that time, I pay for them myself. At $200 a month, I am lucky. Some of us pay a lot more for the chance to be sane.

I believe that, one day, a solution better than three pills a day without a guarantee of sanity will arrive.

I believe that, one day, I will have learned the art of hanging gently.

And I believe that I will have earned it.

And so, I wait. Still, I wait.

Andrea Woodside recently moved from Toronto to London, England.

ON BORDERLINE PERSONALITY DISORDER: We didn't hear from many people with this controversial disorder, but Dianne Stringer wrote this from small-town Ontario.

"Borderlines, I've read and heard, are notoriously difficult to treat and be around. What kept bringing me back to the hospital were self-injurious and suicidal behaviours. Labels were placed upon me and people were less than enthused to deal with me. I was a behavioural problem. Not a human being – a behavioural problem. A patient who'll suck the life out of anyone dumb enough to try helping. The guilt I've carried since first being told of the diagnosis has been a heavy weight. For years I denied its existence. Yet, here I am telling you my story. How strange is that?"

> **ON SELF-INJURY:** Joan Hay (profiled on page 256) describes how, several years ago, in the depths of depression, she would cut her arms.
>
> "Didn't feel it. Didn't hurt. You almost have this other voice saying, 'What are you doing? What's going on?' But I kept cutting. It was such a natural thing to do. So there must be something within us that we get to the point that something has to burst. And it became ritualistic. It'd be the first thing I'd think of when I needed an out. It's a purging and it's very addictive. I would even be in the hospital and I'd go around looking for tabs off of pop cans — anything I could get my hands on. I can't believe that was me."

KIM HONEY
On Panic Attacks

The crushing pain in my chest jolted me out of sleep. I looked at the clock: it was 3 a.m. Waves of terror lapped at my brain, drowning out any rational thought. I curled up in a ball, face down in the single futon, gasping for air. My heart was beating so hard and so fast, I was certain I was dying. My roommate slept on in the bedroom next door, and loath to make a scene, I dragged myself out to the balcony of our eleventh-floor apartment to get some air. I couldn't decide if I was having a heart attack or losing my mind. I had this strange compulsion to throw myself over the railing, even though I am deathly afraid of heights.

It was the middle of December and a snowstorm was raging. My heart was exploding in my chest, and I felt sick to my stomach. It had to be a heart attack. After fifteen, twenty minutes of this hell, I woke up my roommate and asked her to take me to the hospital.

It was after four when we arrived. When the admitting nurse asked me about my symptoms, I reached into my shirt and could still feel my heart hammering in my chest. I was whisked into emergency and hooked up to a heart monitor. The electrode pads were cold, but the sound of my heart thumping out its rhythm and the sight of the spiky line rising and falling in a regular pattern on the screen were soothing. As soon as the doctor hooked me up, I felt an overwhelming sense of calm. My heart was back to normal and the chest pains were gone. I was so utterly exhausted, I fell asleep. They sent me home a few hours later with strict instructions to return if it happened again. It was not unheard of for a thirty-three-year-old woman to have a heart attack.

Something strange had been happening to me ever since I moved to Toronto a few months before. It always happened outside work, and always started with the feeling that I couldn't breathe. It usually happened when I was relaxed, even after a few beers, even in the middle of REM sleep. Some attacks would pounce on me in the middle of the night and I would wake up, terrified, in full fight-or-flight mode. The attacks lasted about five minutes, although some lasted as long as half an hour. At first they seemed to creep up on me, and I wouldn't even realize what was happening until I was gasping for breath. The adrenalin rush was profuse, and it often made me vomit as the attack receded.

Sometimes people were with me when it happened. My face would be ashen, my eyes wide with fear. Once I knew what was happening, I would hide. A bathroom stall was my favourite place to wait one out, because I could put my head between my legs, and if I had to throw up, the toilet was right there. I was embarrassed to tell people what was going on. One friend, who was showing me around her new house when she witnessed me gasping for air at the top of her stairs, told me I was out of shape. I missed a lot of social events because of these episodes, including a friend's wedding ceremony and a football game at the SkyDome.

Along with the attacks came odd symptoms that I brushed aside. I couldn't eat any solid food, because I had an overwhelming fear I would choke to death. Obviously, I lost a lot of weight, about twenty pounds and two dress sizes. My usually mild tendency to claustrophobia became more pronounced. I dreaded going to work, because I was afraid of getting stuck in the elevator, the subway might break down in a tunnel, the power might get cut to the streetcar. In all these phobic scenarios, the underlying theme was that I would suffocate because there wouldn't be enough air.

In time I came to recognize the warning signs: a feeling of dread, bizarre fears, auditory hallucinations (footsteps from a non-existent burglar, for example), an inability to swallow, and, the dead giveaway, no breath.

Six days a week I took the subway, then the streetcar to work at the *Globe and Mail*, where I was a copy editor. Sometimes I had to get off before my stop and wait out an attack before I could get back on. The newsroom was the only place I felt safe. But then, when the next big attack came, it hit me at work. White as a ghost, I stumbled to a friend's desk and told her I couldn't breathe. As instructed, I immediately took a cab to the hospital. This time, they weren't as concerned. Because I was new to the city, they told me to make an appointment at the hospital's clinic. Desperately hoping that someone would finally be able to help me, I showed up a day or two later. I fled in tears after an intern, who told me he was going to take my medical history, asked if I wanted an AIDS test.

The attacks were getting more frequent, more debilitating. Four, five times a day, I would be launched into a dark underworld ruled by maladjusted synapses and neurons, where nothing was certain except the feeling that I was going mad and I was going to die.

Finally I diagnosed myself. I was reading the classified ads in a local magazine when I saw it: "Panic Attacks, Anxiety," it said. "I Can Help." I phoned the number, and talked to a former sufferer long enough to determine that I had, indeed, gone a little crazy. Still, to this day, I blame my panic attacks on wonky neurochemistry. This is the way I picture it: Everyone is born with a gas tank full of serotonin sloshing around inside their brains, but that neurochemical can be depleted by the stresses of life. How badly it's depleted depends on your personality. In my case, I had been seriously depressed for a month before the panic attacks started, ever since the love of my life dumped me and left town. So I needed a little serotonin top-up. Who wouldn't?

A general practitioner finally referred me to a psychiatrist. I remember sitting in his waiting room, looking around at the other patients, surprised to see they all looked normal. I couldn't imagine there was anything wrong with them. I didn't really want to see a shrink, but I was desperate. The minute I walked into his office I burst into tears and didn't stop crying for an hour. I had been terrified for so long, and I was afraid to admit to anyone just how stricken I was.

He offered an antidepressant. I refused, because I thought drugs were for real head cases, and I was obviously still all there. I told him we would talk once a week and see how that went. When he tried to probe my childhood, I lied to him. Not that there was anything to hide. I just didn't want to risk saying something that might interest him enough that he would want to continue seeing me for, say, years. I wanted a quick fix and I would be on my way.

I became more and more discouraged as the weeks wore on and I still wasn't cured. I finally gave in and took Paxil (an antidepressant, also used for anxiety), because the panic attacks weren't getting any better and I couldn't bear to live with them one more minute of the day. I also had Ativan, which were supposed to stop the panic attacks in their tracks, but they never did. They just made me really sleepy. Later, I learned they could, in fact, stave off an attack, but I had to take one as soon as I felt the first pang of anxiety.

It took about two weeks for the Paxil to kick in, and I remember crossing the days off my calendar, waiting for the panic attacks to subside. They eventually did. After three months, I decided I was cured and stopped taking the pills.

It has been five years since my life was consumed by the vagaries of my brain. I realize now that what happened to me was probably exacerbated by my Type A personality. I was always a worrier, I was always impatient and competitive. (Now, and only now, do I remember that I had my first panic attack in high school when I was worrying about passing a math course I desperately needed to get into university. Without a degree, I felt my life would be over.)

In those five years, my world righted itself. The love of my life returned to me; we are married and have a daughter whose company

I cherish; I have a job reporting at the *Globe*, which has fulfilled a life-long goal. And I still suffer the occasional panic attack, about one every two months. This I can live with, although I would rather not, particularly since I now know the triggers intimately: crowds, heights, insects (I am highly allergic to bee stings), and hangovers.

I have also learned that I had a predisposition to this mental illness; my mother suffered from panic attacks, something I didn't know until I described mine to her and she told me the same thing happened to her when she was in her twenties. She was a worrier, too. I suspect that her aunt, my great-aunt Marg, had a version of the same thing, since she always talked about a "ledge" she had in her throat that wouldn't allow her to swallow certain things. So now three generations in my family have had it.

It still doesn't help to know this. I look at my daughter and her beyond-beautiful face and wonder if I've passed on more than just eye colour and mischievousness. I ache for her already. But I have steel in my bones, too, and a vivacious streak, and an appreciation for the smaller things in life, and it all makes my heart sing. Even if she does inherit my addled brain, I figure she'll get some of the good stuff, too.

Kim Honey is a news reporter at the Globe and Mail.

ON POSTTRAUMATIC STRESS DISORDER: (Retired) Lt.-Gen. Roméo Dallaire developed PTSD after a military assignment in Rwanda.

"You become very leery of the dark and the silence. . . . The silence is intolerable . . . It opens up all kinds of opportunities, be they dreams, daydreaming or sitting there with nothing else moving and suddenly, you're back there. . . . Sometimes a word, a statement, a smell, an action, literally throws you into an uncontrolled state. It can be anger, incredible depression. You can be literally unable to function. You do become suicidal and you do do attempts."   — quoted in *Toronto Star*, April 13, 2000

LYNDA WONG
On Anorexia

If you were to ask me five years ago if I thought I'd ever see the light at the end of the tunnel, I probably would have denied ever being in a tunnel. I was mentally and emotionally blinded by my own desires and obsessions. Not aware that I was hurting the people around me, or that I was hurting myself.

My journey into darkness started off innocently, as a self-conscious fourteen-year-old girl just wanting to lose a few pounds. Like anyone, I wanted to be liked by others and accepted by my peers, but my trip took a few unexpected turns. Before long I was lying in a hospital bed hooked up to machines and having fluid pumped into my malnourished, frail little body. I remember my first day in hospital, the doctor looked straight into my emotionless eyes and warned me about this fatal disease and said that without treatment I would die. Her words bounced off of me like ping-pong balls. "*Me*, die? Ha, what does *she* know?"

Over the next year and a half, I became a "revolving-door" patient; weaving in and out of hospital was my specialty. What began with a drive to lose weight ended up as a full-blown eating disorder.

My first experience with hospital food lived up to expectations; it was disgusting. However, it was a lot better than the liquid meal replacement I was given. "Chocolate, strawberry, or vanilla?" – that was the question of the hour, every hour, the three flavours of a milkshake-like meal-replacement drink I would grow to hate more and more each day. "Ensure" was its name. All that mattered to me, though, was that it was food – my greatest foe.

My first choice was strawberry – low-cal, right? My eyes almost popped out of my head when I discovered it had 250 calories per *can*. That's how much I was eating a *week*! Before my hospital admission, I was surviving on half an orange and a small bowl of salad (technically just lettuce with vinegar) a day. This was probably why the easy-to-absorb liquid Ensure was all I was given at first.

During my first admission, I was a model patient, gaining weight steadily and obeying all the rules, which meant eating within the required time limit, attending group-therapy sessions, and never complaining or causing any trouble on the ward. Ten long weeks later, I was thrown back out into the real world, not cured, but at a safe enough weight. My freedom didn't last long (five days to be exact), and there I was, back in the hospital.

This cycle continued for a year, and with each of the next nine admissions, I became increasingly bitter at my parents and at the hospital. In a way, I was determined to keep my eating disorder. The more power the hospital or my parents took away from me, the more I rebelled, trying to regain some control. And if I was going to be forced to stay in the hospital, I could at least make my stay difficult for everyone. Soon my eating disorder began taking on a mind of its own.

When the staff felt I was ready, I was allowed to eat solid food. This was considered a privilege, a step up, I guess you could say. But for me, it was a step down. Solid food was much easier to hide. Even with the nurses watching like a hawk, you'd be surprised how much food I managed to hide while in hospital.

It wasn't so easy with the liquid meal replacement. It seemed every day I was reaching new lows, and one of the most memorable must have been my "sporty outfit" scheme. This consisted of a hockey jersey and a pair of athletic pants. Airy, comfortable hospital attire, right? But I liked it for another quality. Absorbancy. At the end of every meal, the sleeves of my jersey and the thighs of my pants would be drenched with vanilla Ensure. (My choice of vanilla was not based on taste but on the fact that, of the three flavours, it stained the least.) I was rarely caught, but when I was, I was forced to make up an estimated amount of liquid spilled.

It wasn't long, however, before I realized that my vanilla-soaked clothes weren't doing me much good. As I was drinking less (spilling more), I failed to gain the required amount of weight. So I would get bumped up a can. At one point I was "drinking" fourteen cans a day – that's 3,500 calories – and still not gaining weight.

My solution to this problem was clear: cheat the scale. This took some planning. First, the skimpy hospital gown didn't leave much to the imagination; second, the nurse in charge of weighing everybody in the morning was no fool; and lastly, what could I use that would be heavy enough to make a difference on the scale, yet small and compact enough to avoid detection?

Without giving too much away, my plan consisted of really sticky, heavy-duty tape, rolls of coins, a small tube with a cap, and lots of water. It proved to be a successful formula.

The battle to stay out of hospital, however, proved to be much harder work. My weekly doctor's appointments were nerve-racking, as each week I had to add on more weights to make up for the amount I had lost. Sometimes I felt like giving up; the effort I put into going to the doctor's was like getting ready to go into outer space. I had to make sure I had "put on" just enough weight yet not so much as to arouse any suspicion. Precision was the key. It became an art in itself. After every victorious appointment, I felt like celebrating. I was forty pounds (or 30 per cent) below normal weight for my age and height – and should have been back in hospital – but to me that didn't matter. The only thing I cared about was losing more.

Somehow, through all of this, it occurred to me that there was something wrong with my life. I realized that my only friends were fellow patients in situations similar to my own. These were supposed to be the happiest and most carefree years of my life, and all I had to show for them were a few hospital bracelets and a pair of hospital pants. Out of hospital, I found myself constantly thinking about being in the hospital. I often wondered how much longer I had left. I knew it was only a matter of time before my devious plan would fall apart – and it would be either death or another stay in hospital. Luckily, the latter came first.

I became a regular. Not just at one hospital, but at a second, and then a third. A veteran nurse at one hospital told me I was the most stubborn patient she had ever met. It was like music to my ears. I was a successful anorexic, and people were finally acknowledging my hard work!

My hospital-to-hospital cycle ended abruptly when I turned eighteen and, in the eyes of the law, I became an adult. I could no longer be forced into hospital against my will. This was the best news for me, but a nightmare for my parents, and I could see how much I was hurting them. It tore me to pieces to think I was making their lives so difficult.

With every step of my disease, I had relied on others to guide me or tell me what to do. My turning point came when I became aware that I was the only one capable of helping myself. I made up my mind that I was not going to be another statistic and, one bite at a time, with my family supporting me through the rough patches and setbacks (and boy, were there a lot), I gradually made progress.

I can now proudly say that my days of half an orange and a bowl of salad are over. Nowadays, I can eat an orange and a bowl of salad as part of one meal! My nightmarish days of Ensure have ended as well, although maybe one day I'll pick up a can for old times' sake. I now allow myself to eat foods that I once considered forbidden – like cookies, bread, pizza, pasta, and cheese – without giving it a second thought.

The end of my teenage years is fast approaching, and I have continued to move forward, rarely looking back to the time when I feared my struggles would never end. I still battle daily with food – I doubt that will ever disappear – but this is a battle I am now winning. Even if I'm not completely cured, I know there's hope. In all that I've seen and gone through in the past few years, what keeps me going is knowing that somewhere, not too far from where I stand, there *is* light at the end of the tunnel.

Lynda Wong, who also appeared in our first book, is now a full-time university student completing a life sciences degree at the University of Toronto.

ON BULIMIA: Leslie Côté (profiled on page 242) describes how binging and purging was, for her, a futile attempt to control her body and her emotions.

"An anorexic can get control over their body. But as a bulimic, I just couldn't do it. . . . It's as if you've got this wall, and it's not a very strong wall, and it's damming something. And there's water starting to come through one of the holes. And you put your hand here, but then water starts coming out this other hole. So you put your hand there. And you don't have enough hands to cover all the different pressure points. Well, that's kind of how I felt. The eating, the binging, and the purging never quite got me control over my life. It would be just temporary; it was fine for today until something else happened."

DIANE F.
On Schizophrenia

I was born into a house of madness. My mother was mentally ill.

There were signs of trouble before I left the hospital. My mother was convinced that I was not her child. I didn't look like the "right baby" to her. It wasn't until I was in grade school that she finally accepted me as her own child.

What I remember most about my mother was her constant anger. She seemed to be at boiling point almost all the time. People were always plotting against her for some reason or another. She would walk around the house doing chores, muttering comebacks to the people who had done her wrong.

My mother's anger spilled over into her behaviour. She was physically abusive to me and my little brother. We walked on eggshells around her, trying not to draw her fury. We were spanked at least once a day, and often several times a day. Over time, she progressed from using her hand to using a paddle or belt.

My father never intervened. He was a preacher and would leave for the office before we woke up, come home for a quick bite, go back out again. In the evenings, he had shut-ins to visit, or hospital calls to make, or meetings with the deacons. In his free time, he worked on his Ph.D. He stayed very busy and very much away from the house.

My brother and I were too young to know that our mother was ill. In fact, it wasn't until I was about twelve that I realized our family was different from others. By the time I entered junior high, the beatings had increased in severity. I was constantly covered in bruises, on my shoulders, back, buttocks, and down the back of my legs. I was suicidal. Although I didn't really want to die; I just wanted the hurting to stop. I could have killed myself, but I couldn't leave my little brother behind. And I didn't see any solution.

Once, I was called into the school counsellor's office, and I hesitantly revealed that my mother spanked me sometimes. The counsellor called my mother and confronted her. That afternoon, my mother held a knife to my throat and told me if I ever told anyone about being beaten again, she would kill me. I believed her.

Then one day, as I was taking the trash to the alley, I heard two men talking about me. "Look how strong she is. She has very muscular legs." I looked around, but I didn't see anyone. The voices kept commenting about what a good runner I would be. I went back inside and thought about this for a while and figured out that the voices were coming from somewhere remote. They had to be Russian agents using advanced technology to spy on me.

I began hearing the Russian agents almost everywhere I went. They were going to kidnap me and take me back to Russia to train for their Olympic track team. This was the seventies, at the height of the Cold War. From what I knew, Russia was a cold, dismal place to live. But on the other hand, it would be a relief to be taken away from my mother.

Over the next few months the voices faded and I began to realize that what I had experienced was not real. My one hope throughout high school was that when I turned eighteen, I could leave home and go to college. I thought that once I left the madness of my home, I would be okay. I could finally be my own person.

I graduated with honours, and in college took pre-med courses, started dating, and was amazed to discover that some of the boys found me attractive. I was so happy to be away from home and all the chaos.

During my second semester, I went on an out-of-town trip with my boyfriend. As we were driving back home, I started seeing animals leaping out in front of the car. A few weeks later, I was walking on campus and saw people in front of me suddenly disappear. One moment they would be there, then they would simply fade from view. About the same time, I lost my ability to concentrate on my studies. No matter how many times I would read a paragraph, I could not retain the information. My grades plummeted.

I knew I was in trouble. I knew that visual hallucinations were not something most people experienced. Reasoning that maybe the stress under which I had grown up was coming back to haunt me, I finally went to the psychology department of the university, where I was introduced to a kind psychologist. I told her I had some problems dealing with my mother, and that I was having hallucinations. She looked at me sadly and told me she couldn't help. She gave me a referral to the local mental health clinic.

The clinic was located on the bad side of town. There were several people outside the building either sleeping or passed out. Inside, the place was in disarray. I was led into a small room and asked questions such as "Do you know where you are? Who is the president? What year is it?" They had some IQ questions as well. Then they started asking me about my upbringing. I gave them a few details. I told them about the hallucinations.

A week later, I met with the psychiatrist, who told me I had a "thought disorder" and wrote me a prescription. He wanted to have some lab tests done to check my thyroid. Well, I didn't have any money to pay for the lab tests. I knew something pretty serious was going on, but I wasn't going back there again. I had decided I would deal with it on my own.

The next summer, I got a job working at a pizza restaurant and met my future husband. Danny was a bright and handsome young man, the assistant manager at the restaurant. We spent every waking hour together, and by the fall we were engaged. I didn't tell Danny much about my mental health problems. I thought they were finally behind me. I did tell him about my mother, and the abuse I had suffered.

We were married around Christmas that year. I couldn't have been happier. Aside from an occasional nightmare about my childhood, I was symptom-free for long stretches of time. I got pregnant about six months after we married. I was overjoyed! I had always wanted children. I just knew things would be different with my children. I would be a good mother to them. They would grow up healthy and happy. Alex was born after an easy delivery. Ben was born two years later.

I managed to finish college eight years after beginning, going to school when I could, and graduating with a degree in medical technology. I passed a national certification exam and had a licence to work in a medical laboratory. Our financial picture greatly improved. My children grew happy and healthy. I did not abuse them. I was a good mother to them. I felt complete.

But things were not so good between me and my husband. For five years, he was only marginally employed, and we had arguments over this. I began having nightmares more often. A common theme would be that my mother was beating me. Sometimes at night, I would pound my fists into Danny, defending myself against my attacker in my sleep.

I began having problems in the daytime, too. Sometimes I would see stars falling from the sky like confetti. Other times, trees would become ominous figures that would bend down towards me as if to devour me. The voices started up again. "Your children are dead. You killed them. Burn in hell, bitch. You are going to die."

At work, I was unable to concentrate. The voices kept distracting me. Beakers and test tubes would move around on the bench independently. I would take frequent breaks, walking around outside to clear my head. The cool air sometimes helped.

Things continued to deteriorate as I gathered courage to seek help. I was having almost constant visual hallucinations, to the point that it was sometimes difficult to see. It looked like it was snowing black snowflakes indoors. Driving to work was a challenge as I struggled to see the road.

I became paranoid at work. Any time two people were talking to each other, I was sure they were talking about me. Everyone hated me. I hated me. I wanted to die.

I finally made an appointment to see a psychologist. I was absolutely terrified of everything at this point, especially going for that first visit.

But the psychologist was very gentle and soft-spoken. I told her that I was having some problems dealing with my past. I didn't mention that I could hardly see her face for all the visual interferences I was having. I don't recall what she said to me, because I was hearing the voices shouting at me throughout the session. But afterwards, I felt more relaxed.

Bit by bit I told her my story. Sometimes I would be so distracted by the voices that I would appear to "blank out" for minutes at a time. This confused her. So she had me come in for some psychological testing. The tests showed that I had a "thought disorder." I asked her what that meant. She explained that a thought disorder could be an illness like schizophrenia or severe depression. She said it was time for me to see a psychiatrist for medication.

When I went to the psychiatrist, I chose against medication, thinking my problems were due to bad parenting and could be taken care of with talk therapy. But I was getting no better. One evening at work, the voices started commanding me to kill myself. "Die, die, die! Die NOW!" I was in a panic. I had to do something. I called my psychologist and was hospitalized that very night.

While I was in the hospital, I was put on an antipsychotic medication. The voices diminished, the visual hallucinations decreased.

I went back to work and continued to improve over time. But one day, I made a simple error and was fired. I was devastated. My husband was not working and I was providing the only income. We had no savings. I had to apply for unemployment and food stamps. I was so ashamed.

Almost immediately, the symptoms returned. Soon, I was almost too sick to look for work. My medications were doubled, then quadrupled, but didn't seem to have any effect. We were about a month away from losing our house. Almost too late, I was able to find a new job, but I was in pretty bad shape. I would try to do the work, but no matter how hard I tried to concentrate, I would mess things up. After six months, they terminated me. But I was not out of work for long this time. The people at my new job were very kind. There was a sort of family atmosphere there.

I made a trip back home to my parents' house. I had not been back in over ten years. It was good to see my father and grandparents again.

But towards the end of my visit, my mother's old pattern of behaviour emerged again and I started suffering a relapse. I made it home and was put back in the hospital.

When I came back to work a few weeks later, the manager took me aside and told me she was proud of me for taking charge of my life. I was pretty sure she didn't know what my hospitalization had been about – I had not told them I had schizophrenia when I interviewed for the job.

That day, I took a big risk and told her that I had a mental illness. She said she hoped I was feeling better and told me I could go back to my job with no change in my responsibilities. I was so relieved.

About a year later, I discovered my husband was having an affair. We separated. I was seeing a new psychologist at this time who recognized the role my family played in my relapses. She also recognized that stress was a big predictor of a relapse. A lot of my time in therapy was devoted to dealing with the abuse I suffered while growing up.

Over time, the nightmares decreased. And the frequency and severity of my psychotic episodes have decreased as well.

Last year, my mother was formally diagnosed with schizophrenia, hospitalized, and put on antipsychotic medication. This should have happened forty years ago.

For years, I thought that my schizophrenia was caused by bad parenting. It wasn't until recently that I came to understand that schizophrenia is an inheritable illness. Certainly, the stress caused many of my relapses, but I probably would have developed schizophrenia regardless of my upbringing.

Today, I am doing well. It has been three years since my last hospitalization. I have minor relapses from time to time, but they are usually due to stress. By talking through the problem and adjusting my medications, I have managed to stay out of hospital and retain custody of my two sons. I am still employed and have a wonderful relationship with my manager, who has been so supportive of me throughout my years there.

I will likely be on medications for the rest of my life, but the side effects are tolerable now. My support team includes my psychologist, psychiatrist, friends, co-workers, and children. It is a winning combination. Life is good again.

Diane F. is our "foreign correspondent," as she lives in the United States and contacted us through a schizophrenia Web site. Since writing this story, she has been hospitalized briefly, but she tells us she's now doing well and has returned to full-time work.

ON ECT: Jim Ross from Toronto is a man in his fifties who suffers from depression. He describes his experience with electroconvulsive therapy.

"You put on hospital garb and climb into one of the beds lined up outside the procedure room. On my visits, usually I was one of six, and, surprisingly, the rest were all ladies. . . . When your time comes, you are wheeled into the treatment room, gel is placed on both temples, and an IV needle is inserted in your arm for the anesthetic. The anesthetic is very short-acting (three minutes or so) and is combined with a muscle relaxant. Just as you drift off, a strap with the contact points is put around your head like a bandana. Before you know it, you wake up in the next room, are fed breakfast, and after your blood pressure is taken you are allowed to go in about an hour. The ECT procedure is totally painless. . . . Some of my 'early-morning group' swore by the procedure, but for me *nothing changed*."

REVEREND ISABELLA ROSS[*]
On Depression

I have had chronic major depression for thirty years. If I asked myself what percentage of my life I have been sick, I'd say between 60 and 70 per cent. From the time I was a little kid, I was maybe not depressed but

---

[*] The name Isabella Ross is a pseudonym.

really anxious; I remember always worrying whether my heart was going to stop beating, and being more consumed with death than kids usually are. And I think maybe that was the beginning of the depression.

My journey to medical help was a long and tortuous one; I didn't get any treatment until I was in my thirties. Since that time, I have been in the hospital maybe five times and have received many, if not all, of the antidepressant medications on the market, as well as mood stabilizers, anti-anxiety and antipsychotic meds, and close to fifty treatments of ECT. I have been in psychotherapy for fifteen years, and I currently see my psychiatrist once a week.

As I write this history down, it surprises me how I have managed to keep it together for all this time, raising a family, working full-time, and finding some enjoyment in life. My doctor tells me that most of the people he sees with illnesses as severe as mine are on long-term disability. I'm glad I am able to just keep on going. When I have to actually get up and lead a service, I can do it, but it does take a huge toll. The energy I have to put into it when I'm sick is ten times the amount I put into it when I'm well.

I have sought, in times of clarity, to gain a sense of how my illness has contributed to my understanding of life, and how it has enriched my life. This is easy to say right now, when I am experiencing a few weeks of remission. When I'm really ill, I hear what's like a tape recorder in my head saying really horrible negative things: *Your life isn't worth anything. It would be better if you weren't here any more. You're destroying other people's lives. You're worthless.* That's what consumes me. I don't have any ability to shut it off.

When I'm really ill, I have a great need to connect with people and say, "I'm not well, please understand," but all the time I'm hearing in the back of my mind: *She hears you, but she doesn't care.* It's like this other voice – I describe it as an invisible wall separating me from other people. And that's the horrible, insidious thing about this illness. It cuts you off from people when you need them the most.

In each year, I experience about three months free of symptoms. Usually I hit a low point in February but I have discovered that this illness has a life of its own. "I walk around by myself most of the time," I wrote in my journal on February 15 last year. "Alone, talking in my head, a running dialogue. I have tried to do something today but each something has slipped a little." Then, a few weeks later: "This day, there are no tapes playing, only clarity. Each step seems a step forward, no longer putting one foot in front of the other. I can hear the birds."

And this pattern recurs; the illness and the slow recovery, the illness and maybe another recovery. It is like living in the same house with a few rooms you know well.

Perhaps the most devastating result of this illness is the effect it has on relationships. I have very few friends, mostly because I am usually ill to some degree. I don't return their calls and the last thing I want is to see other people when I am depressed. The anticipation of talking is endless agony.

My friends Jean and Bob understand the most. When I am ill, they listen, hear, and when I say I need them, they say they would like to see me. Pure grace. When I am in the hospital one of them visits every day, and we walk the halls together, sometimes holding hands. They love me and I love them. My doctor does the same sort of thing, in a doctor type of way. He accompanies, listens, hears, suggests, and encourages. He is a warm, caring human being whom I trust. There are few physicians as skilled and caring as he.

My immediate family have lived through the ravages of anger, unpredictability, silence, and discontent. I love them and they love me. My husband tries to be as supportive as he can, but he can come in only so far. The important thing is that he's never gone anywhere; he's remained a constant. With my children, I've always tried to be very honest and describe to the best of my ability what's happening. One of my big worries was always that they would get sick. I'm sure it's been very hard for them when I haven't been well, but I don't know if they could describe it, because it's just something that they grew up with. I think they probably have a lot of knowledge and an awareness that they can't articulate right now. I don't know, they seem okay.

I am aware that because I have "success" – a job, a home, a family, love, and mutual companionship – that this has made it easier. But I have experienced my share of scorn and rejection. For example, in the emergency room of a hospital, because I could walk and talk, some of the triage nurses treated me with open contempt, saying, "Oh, it's you again" on my second visit in a year, and directing me to the "quiet room," where people in the know walk by and give you that look. Blood brings care; tears bring avoidance.

One of the worst "side effects" I've had is memory loss, from the ECT, I guess. The actual procedure is really not anything; the worst part is waiting to have it, the anticipation of it, the thought of what's going on, if it's going to affect my brain in some way. The biggest thing for me is that I've lost a lot of my long-term memory. My husband will say to me, "Remember when we went with the kids to Quebec?" Blank. Absolutely blank. Not even anything at the back of my head. Gone. And I'm convinced that it is the ECT that's done it. I guess the bottom line is that it is worth it, though, because it's helped me to get better. But it's not ideal, and it's the last thing I choose. The thought of it, even after all these treatments, is just awful. But maybe it's actually saved my life. When I look back on it, maybe it has. So I guess in some ways I'm thankful. With all the medications I've taken, you get to the end of what can be done.

For a long time, I felt the ministry might be the place for me, but I held back because when I was sick I thought *I'm not good enough to do that job, I can't really do it*. And then at forty-five, ten years after I graduated (with a Master of Divinity from the University of Toronto), I just decided I was going to do it now or never. In the end, people in the church were almost totally supportive. They said, "This depression has informed who you are as a person. You have learned a huge amount about empathy, about caring for other people because of that illness. And look at it in some ways as . . . a gift is not the right word . . . as what you bring to the ministry." On a really basic level, I'm not fearful of people with mental illness. I feel very connected to them, very comfortable with everything around mental illness. And for that I am very thankful, because in this kind of work you come up against it a lot. It's also given me a lot more compassion for people with illnesses. It's given me a great understanding of being a companion, of just staying with a person, of not expecting miraculous results. It's more just travelling along with them. And that's been a great gift to me.

I don't think God sends illnesses or takes them away. But I certainly see the presence of God in every illness. Not just mental illness, in *every* illness. And in the connection that's made between people in times when they are vulnerable, in times when their needs are greater. I think it draws out in the other person their own sense of vulnerability, and then there's a sharing that goes on at a different level than in a regular relationship. I certainly see the presence of God in that.

I will probably always know depression, but it surprises me, each time I am in recovery, how far off the depression can seem and how hard it is to recall the symptoms. That, I imagine, is the blessing of health. When you are sick, you can't imagine what it is like to be well; when you are well, you can't imagine that you were really sick. And I appreciate so much when I am well. To me, it means being able to live in the present, not being haunted by fear all the time, not having your mind overrun with negative thoughts. It's feeling connected to other people. Being well is not this great euphoria or happiness; it's sort of waking up in the morning and knowing what to expect.

When I'm well I think, "If only I could stay like this for the rest of my life." But in reality, that has not been my experience. Recovery is, the way I describe it, a few months of living in the light. But you always hope. You *always* have this hope that it might be for the rest of your life.

Reverend Isabella Ross is a United Church minister in Toronto.

ON STIGMA: Kelly is a young woman from B.C., recently diagnosed with bipolar disorder, who wrote to us about the dilemmas posed by stigma.

"It's not easy. I want to go back to work, get on with my life, but I feel like everything about me is tainted now. I feel useless and broken and nervous that I'm now stamped for life with the mark of the 'other.' How do you explain this to someone? How do you tell prospective employers that you had this little run-in with mental illness – but you're much better now? How do you get your brain around the fact that your 'severe illness' has symptoms that include increased sex drive, eloquence, charisma, elation, and shopping? I mean, SHOPPING, for God's sake? Really, it makes you feel a little silly and sheepish."

JANE LOWRY
On Postpartum Mental Illness

Postpartum psychosis must be the most cruel, twisted joke Mother Nature could ever play, and probably on the list of the world's best-kept secrets. The miracle of birth – the time in one's life that is supposed to be full of a never-before-experienced kind of joy – instead can turn into something beyond one's worst imaginable nightmare.

I had been rather over-protective since my first child was born, never away for more than a few hours at a time, never making any attempt to find a babysitter, and even apprehensive about leaving him with his own father, knowing that he was not as attentive as I. Although I did have the "luxury" of being a stay-at-home mom, I did not have the luxury of nimble grandparents available at the drop of a hat.

After my second child was born, my over-protective behaviour escalated into suspiciousness. Then one day it turned to full-blown paranoia, and my husband's cousin Judy, a physiotherapist, insisted I go into the hospital that night to see someone. Since I'm almost always an agreeable person, I agreed to go to the hospital along with Judy, but first we had to establish that our house was still intact and my parents hadn't been murdered, as I had feared was scheduled to also happen that evening. My husband then watched me fairly calmly pack up some valuables and clothing as if we would never return to our house again. I even left a message with our insurance company telling them that I wasn't sure the house would exist much longer, as I had felt threatened via the Internet that it was to be blown up. I also wanted to call the police and warn the neighbours, but I was discouraged from doing this.

My answers to the emergency-room doctor's questions convinced him that I must stay for forty-eight hours. I had made reference to Dr. Suzanne Killinger-Johnson, mentioning something about how one never knows what one will do if one is upset. [In Toronto a few months earlier, Suzanne Killinger-Johnson had jumped in front of a subway train with her baby in her arms. Both died. She was suffering from postpartum depression.] Little did I know that I was suffering from a similar disorder. I told them that I felt fine, and that what I had feared hadn't happened, so there was nothing to worry about. I figured, wrongly, I could just go home then.

It was about 3 a.m., New Year's morning 2001, and I began to feel absolute fear there in the hospital.

My five-month-old baby wasn't allowed to stay with me. If I had known this, I would never have set foot in the building. I was nursing, and she had never been away from me before. The insensitive nurse (I have the utmost respect and admiration for nurses, my mom being a retired one) said the baby was old enough to stop breast-feeding anyway. She had also told Judy that I couldn't be suffering from a postpartum disorder because my baby was already too old. She didn't seem to know that various forms of mental illness can surprise a potentially vulnerable mom months after she's given birth.

I declined the offer of medication that would supposedly help "clear my thoughts." I had to keep all my wits about me if I was going to survive this place, and I thought the medication would likely confuse me or kill me. The sign on the door of my assigned room said "BED A" and directly under that, "BED B." I quickly rearranged the letters in my head to spell out "BE DEAD," with a couple of letters left over that didn't matter. I doubted that any of the doctors were real doctors, and the nurses didn't seem like real nurses. In fact, even the patients seemed as if they were reading lines from a script, saying things that were intended to shock me or work on my mind to make it snap.

There were no phones in the rooms, and the pay phone didn't give me change from my dollar coin for the single call I made. Another intimidation tactic, no doubt. I kept the few quarters I had in my sock, convinced that once they were used up, I would be cut off from the outside world forever. And surely they were going to poison my food; I tried to consume only things in closed containers, such as yoghurt, milk, or juice.

A psychiatrist diagnosed me with postpartum depression, although I didn't feel at all depressed and had no symptoms of depression. I was simply more terrified than I'd ever imagined possible. I was sure the diagnosis had been cleverly fabricated to keep me there so they could kill me. I told him I felt fine. I smiled and joked that my husband had been home for three months on parental leave, and that was probably what had driven me crazy.

Many little things convinced me that there was a large Nazi conspiracy at work, and I was on their list to be eliminated. Someone came to take a blood sample from me. I was sure the needle was infected with AIDS, since they had failed to poison my food or make me snap. A nurse who came to take my blood pressure said, "You couldn't be any more normal if you tried." I smiled. I was sure she was one of *them*, and that she knew I was absolutely terrified but hiding it.

Yet I was allowed to check out of "Hotel California" after spending two nights. Happy New Year. My survival instincts had been fully activated, but were actually working against me. I should undoubtedly have been kept in there and put on medication immediately, but somehow I had been able to convince everyone I was perfectly fine, and since my house hadn't blown up, I could indeed go home.

Over the next six months, my mind created many worst-case scenarios and then methodically, one by one, took me through them, convincing me that each delusion was completely real. It was as if terrorists had hijacked my mind. I was dodging Nazis, police, and death every day. I was under twenty-four-hour surveillance with the latest in satellite technology, which meant my every action and word was monitored. *They* could see through the walls of our house. I was a prisoner.

I was often certain that my husband and his entire family were part of the Nazi plot because of their Austrian background (same as Hitler). I had to rely on myself to survive, and to save the world. A tall order for a stay-at-home mom. I considered contacting the RCMP and other international intelligence organizations, but knew that the spies would see what I was attempting to do and intercept my calls, or strategically place their own people to handle my report.

I was able to see that my thoughts were far-fetched, but nothing anyone said could convince me they were not real, so I stopped talking about them. I was determined to survive as long as possible to look after my children, and amazingly I was able to take my son to preschool, attend birthday parties, shovel snow, make dinner, do laundry as if nothing were really all that wrong. The usual daily multi-tasking, but with an added psychotic twist.

I talked to my imaginary spy people, asked them questions about what was going to happen to me and who exactly they were. They gave me answers via licence plates and media sources. I drove my car to places where I thought I was supposed to meet someone who would kill me, even though I didn't want to die. The scary thing being that I took my baby with me each time, thinking that somehow *they* couldn't kill a mom with a baby, like not hitting a guy wearing glasses. I was very lucky not to have had any accidents, as I tried to read every licence plate within sight every time I went out, convinced they could provide me with clues.

The spies were always there, always polite, always subtle, but never harmful. A typical example was a sweet elderly gentleman who approached me in the grocery-store aisle and informed me that if his wife were there, she would want to steal such a cute baby. I managed a smile.

I had been trying to thwart all efforts to get me on medication for fear it would kill me. The one prescribed was called Zyprexa, and when I rearranged the letters, it spelled RAPE XYZ. I assumed it was a scary name for a phony drug fabricated especially to kill me.

I finally gave in and started taking the medication in May after friends contacted the mobile crisis people, who diplomatically convinced me that medication was better than the hospital. I had to agree with them on that one (although later I would note that the hospital was a much more agreeable and harmless place than I had originally thought it was).

I rarely even took Aspirin, and the thought that I would be on an "antipsychotic" seemed ridiculous. I was not sick. But I had become careless, letting slip a few too many details of what was on my mind.

I made sure my husband was witness as I took each low-dose pill. The medication seemed to dull the licence-plate messages a bit, and I did sleep much more deeply, although it was harder to get up in the morning. I abruptly decided on my own to stop taking it after thirty-three days, with seven pills left. I was still paranoid that the last pill would be the one to deliver the final lethal bit of whatever it was I was being slowly poisoned with. I still held on to a tiny strand of hope that something would foil *their* plans, and by some fluke I would be allowed to live.

I had not been brought up with religion, but one evening I decided to talk to God. I told Him I was sorry I hadn't talked to Him sooner. I told Him that since I felt I was under constant surveillance and had no privacy, I had not felt comfortable talking to Him and that I only wanted to talk to Him in private. The next day, as if a magic spell were broken, I suddenly realized that the fears that had plagued me for months were not at all real. It came as quite the shock. As time passed, I felt better and better. In a bizarre coincidence, the day I snapped out of it was the day Andrea Yates drowned her children.

Had God helped me? I like to think so. I hope He will help her, too.

It was as if my mind had been cleansed. I went back on the Internet and did some research on postpartum depression. To my surprise, I stumbled upon postpartum psychosis. My case was not the mildest, nor was it the worst. No one had even mentioned it to me.

I remember how clearly it had been imprinted in my mind during prenatal class that there were some very remote chances, possibly one in a zillion, that one could become paralyzed or suffer some other severe side effect from having an epidural. I remember the entire pre-natal class made one big list of all our fears, such as something being wrong with the baby or a difficult delivery. No one told me that becoming pregnant put me in the running to completely lose my mind as a result of haywire hormones. If postpartum psychosis were not such a "shhhh, don't scare the pregnant women" issue, the potentially vulnerable one-in-a-thousand mothers who endure it would have a better chance of receiving proper treatment right away and avoiding an experience like mine.

My second child was only eleven days old when Dr. Killinger-Johnson's postpartum disorder led her to an escape route. I was as shocked as everyone else. Not any more. I completely understand how the mind could conclude such a thing was a logical and necessary action.

The depths of the mind that I have delved into, and the power of the mind that I have seen first-hand, fascinate me. I have an understanding of things I never dreamed I'd understand. Unpleasant as it was at the time, the further away from it I get, the more confident I am in saying that it was truly one of the best things that has ever happened to me.

I volunteer my story wholeheartedly for Dr. Suzanne Killinger-Johnson, her baby Cuyler, for Andrea Yates, for their families and friends, and for all mothers who have suffered postpartum depression with the hope that people will get talking about mental illnesses, whether postpartum or otherwise.

Jane Lowry is a stay-at-home mom who is pursuing volunteer work in the field of mental health.

ON OBSESSIVE-COMPULSIVE DISORDER (OCD): Jane (a pseudonym) is a psychology student at Concordia University in Montreal. She has recovered with the help of cognitive-behavioural therapy, and hopes to become a psychologist specializing in OCD.

"The disorder started with classic symptoms, which began when I was seventeen, while I was still attending [high school]. I was constantly obsessing that I had done something wrong. This was complicated by rituals; unless I did them, something bad would happen. It was very difficult for me to concentrate on schoolwork. I started checking: when I left my house, I thought I had left the garage door open, [or] some appliance was somehow going to malfunction and become dangerous. Once, when I was driving, I thought that I had hit someone and couldn't get that thought out of my mind. I even had someone take me back to the place where I had driven. After that, I did not drive for almost three years. These thoughts and compulsions left me crying in confusion. I was frightened to do many things on my own, because I might do something wrong when, in reality, I had never done anything 'bad' in my life."

KAREN BOND
On a Daughter's Plight

We always knew my mother had lots of energy, was eccentric, and had a dramatic personality. What we did not know was that she had bipolar disorder, and that the lack of social services and aid would eventually kill her.

I am the youngest of four children, and about ten years ago, when I was twenty-three and my mom was in her early sixties, my sister and I noticed that our slightly outrageous mother was acting more so than usual. Spending excessively, drinking excessively, all the signs that we now know are so common.

One of the first clues was when she made an afternoon visit to our home. After a somewhat frenzied visit that had lasted only a matter of minutes, she was gone. She left behind the plastic cup she had brought in from her car. I went to throw it out and was overwhelmed by the reek of alcohol. The cup was filled with vodka and just a dash of OJ. We were very surprised, because she rarely drank. Before we could stop her, she peeled down the quiet street, and all we could do was hope that she made it home without hurting herself or someone else.

Soon, she was moving back and forth from Toronto to Florida several times each year. With less than a few days' notice, she would prevail on my sister and me to arrange it all, and we would. At any given time, she would arrive back in town and be waiting in one of our apartments when we got home from work. Later, we discovered that she was criminally charged several times in the States for drinking and driving, stalking, and willfully damaging someone's car. This explained the sudden returns to Canada.

I've lost count of the number of times people blamed us kids. Or the times the phone rang and a complete stranger (on one memorable occasion a bellhop from California!) told me to be nicer to my mother. Truly, had you ever seen my tiny, beautiful mother, she and her mania would have charmed the pants off you. She was university-educated and very well-read. Slim, fit, and always well-dressed, with a dangling cigarette and toss of her head she could put you in mind of Bette Davis.

We spent years cleaning up the aftermath of her behaviour – including closing down a consignment store she had opened on a whim and filled with her own clothes – having her live with us in our one-bedroom apartments after she had backed herself into yet another corner. And then our Visa cards would go missing and our phone bills would be $500, and off she'd go for months, leaving us with the guilty relief that, finally, there was a break.

At one particularly bad point, she had rented a two-bedroom apartment on the street where my sister and I lived. She had decided to rent out not one but both bedrooms to total strangers. She slept on a couch in the living room. One of the roommates was a young female university student, who happened to be Jewish. Before I knew it, we were getting visits from this girl who was making serious allegations. She told us that my mom had kicked her out, sold her stuff, and was sending anti-Semitic hate mail to her new address. Sadly, we knew she was probably telling the truth.

Eventually the abuse got so bad, charges were pressed, and my mom, who was sixty-six years old at the time, was to appear in court. I took the day off work to go, hoping I could convince a judge that my mom needed to be forced to get some sort of psychiatric assessment.

In many instances, the police had been involved, and they had told us to go to a doctor or a justice of the peace in order to get some action. We had already tried without success to get a doctor to sign the form for an involuntary assessment.

I could not find my mom in court that day but managed to get in to see a justice of the peace. When I mentioned my mom's name, he commented that someone else had been in that same morning trying to have her "locked up." It turned out to be the student who'd rented a room from my mother. I started crying as I described her actions of late: many menacing calls, hate mail to us and to the student, drunk driving, and vandalism to my car. He became very agitated when I got emotional, and very brusquely told me to stop crying. I could not. Instead, my voice raised a pitch and I began pleading with him, explaining that we had tried several ways to get help for my mom. He kept insisting that there was nothing he could do. I pointed out to him that if, in one day, two people had seen him about the disturbing mental state of someone, maybe he'd better take note. I guess he didn't like my tone, because he promptly had me thrown out of his office.

My mother would be fine for long stretches of time and then would have what we termed "episodes." We began to think that she was a psychopath, as she appeared to have no remorse. When she was "well," she refused to get help, just shrugging it all off.

It seemed endless. No one would help, and we didn't know what to do. Police kept treating the incidents as domestic violence. My sister and I could not, as our other siblings did, write her off and refuse to see her. She was our mother, for heaven's sake. When we were growing up, she held down full-time jobs and managed both a home and a cottage with no help from our dad. She held dinner parties for my father's business associates, played bridge, and ensured that all four kids were involved in sports and music. We knew that life with my alcoholic father had not been easy for her, and we had supported her when she divorced him.

In many respects, she was a fabulous role model for her children. She was the only one of her family to get a higher education and to marry well. She had multiple careers, as a teacher, accountant, office manager, and legal secretary. She was the only girl in her family who married a non-Italian. My dad was a vice-president with a big salary, and our lives were filled with tennis clubs, an Olympic-sized swimming pool at home, and family trips to Bermuda. It tore us up when we'd see her now, with wild hair and shoddy clothes, looking like a bag lady.

It was tough for people to understand. Most said, Oh, everyone's mom/family/sister is a bit weird. People who met her would say she was just a little eccentric. We sisters have a saying: No one knows what it's like to be Mary's children except Mary's children.

The telephone became her weapon. She would call my places of work and talk endlessly to co-workers about our family. Some colleagues were understanding, most made hurtful jokes. It was so embarrassing to walk into work and have someone smirk and say, "Your mom called and kept me on the phone for an hour. Boy, I didn't know you had such an interesting family!" I would turn red, and that familiar helpless feeling would wash over me. What had she said? How bad had she been? I usually didn't ask, because I simply didn't want to know. And, sadly, sometimes I would try to joke back in an effort to cope with the humiliation.

The situation finally came to a head. We had not heard from my mom in many months, and I had even considered calling a private detective in Florida to try to track her down. I could not shake the image of her living as a street person, alone and unable to reach out to us for help.

Then back she came, and we found her a bachelor apartment and moved her in, again. Within a couple of weeks she rapidly deteriorated. She tried to kill herself twice. Finally, my aunt found a doctor who agreed to commit her and she spent three weeks in a psychiatric hospital.

When she had been released only a few weeks and was doing well on medication, she contracted pneumonia. It was then that the doctors noticed the damage to her heart. They were amazed she had never experienced a heart attack. She probably had, but was so far gone she didn't even realize it.

She was sent home after five days, and about a week later, I went to her apartment to give her a bath. It was two days after my thirty-first birthday. I walked in to silence; my mother was lying still on her bed. She had died in her sleep.

We can only guess at what kind of relationship we might have had with her, now that she had finally been diagnosed and was being properly treated. The day before she died, she told my sister that she wanted to get physically better to help with her newborn grand-daughter. I'm glad she didn't know her time was over, and I am grateful that she had attained some sort of peace before she died.

The entire experience has marred my family. My brother moved to the other side of the earth, literally, and has not been in touch for over five years. He refuses to communicate. My sister deals with the guilt of not wanting my mother to know where she lived. (I was the only one of my mom's children not to change phone numbers in case she should need me.) We are still trying to repair our relationship.

I work in the publishing world, and am surrounded by liberal thinkers. They might disagree with me, but what I hope for is a balance between forced medication and opportunities for people to go for help. Manic people cannot do it for themselves, and the way the system works now, neither can their families. I know that, had my mother gotten proper treatment earlier, she would have lived longer and enjoyed a better life.

I don't want the white vans to roll up and cart some poor un-suspecting sod off the street and inject him because the government is taking medicating the mentally ill into their own hands. But you know what? I wish I'd met a doctor who understood what it was like to have an insane person ruling your life. I wish just one doctor could have had the courage to send her in for an involuntary assessment. I'd love to tell that justice of the peace, equipped with the knowledge I have now, "Yes, I'm crying and emotional, but do you know the hell I am living through?" Maybe someone should teach him some compassion.

I am amazed that the actions, often criminal, of an elderly lady were not enough to cause concern. I suppose if she'd killed someone during a drunk-driving spree, someone might have stepped in. I went to the police, to doctors, even to hospital counsellors, and no one seemed sure of what to do.

Since her death I have talked openly about my mom and have done my best to draw a realistic picture of her illness and the effects it had on our family. I am discovering that almost everyone I speak to knows someone who has some form of mental illness. I am no longer ashamed. I will keep my mother's memory alive by remembering the good and the bad, and by forgiving her for what she had no control over.

Karen Bond works as a production manager in the magazine industry.

ON CRACK ADDICTION: Rachael (a pseudonym), a young woman from Toronto, who has been "clean" for several months now, remembers the day she went from hanging out with crack users to actually becoming one at the age of fifteen.

"I was so curious about the high. Everybody in that place smoked crack, or sold crack. So after hanging around there for a few months, I was just totally curious. That day, I got the money, went back to the [crack house], got the crack . . . and it felt *so* good. I felt so energetic. I felt like I could do *anything*. The power of it! It goes straight to your head. It's an upper. It keeps you awake, you lose your appetite. You just feel really good when you inhale the smoke."

SUE GOODWIN
On Surviving Suicide and Poverty

Sue Goodwin left work one day with a simple, spontaneous plan: She intended to die. Midway through a regular shift in a regular office, she walked calmly into a Toronto subway station. The young woman proceeded downstairs and positioned herself on the edge of the platform. Then she waited for the telltale blast of air and the glare of approaching headlights. It was February 26, 1986.

"I remember standing on the platform, thinking, 'This will show all the people who've hurt me. This will show them what they've done to me.'" The rush of air was coming. The train hurtled toward the station. "And then I jumped." The lead car slammed into her back at full speed, shattering nearly every rib along her spine and pulverizing two vertebrae. Her right leg cracked apart. Her head hit the train, then the ground. For a very long time, everything was black. The coma lasted five weeks; it would be three months before she regained a state of mind resembling what most of us would deem conscious thought. [*]

This is Sue's story.

I tried to commit suicide because I thought nobody loved me, because of what happened to me when I was a kid.

My adoptive parents split up when I was seven and divorced when I was nine, so I was part of a custody war. Unfortunately, the court decided in favour of my mother. I don't think she ever wanted kids, so I don't know why she fought so hard to have us. A man who was close to my family started coming over; I didn't like him, I didn't trust him, and not surprisingly, there was a good reason for that. He sexually abused me from the time I was nine until I left home because of it, the day after I turned sixteen.

I waited until I was in my twenties to search for my birth parents. The Children's Aid Society told me my dad was manic-depressive and my mom had to quit high school to have me. But I think my life would have gone just tickety-boo if it weren't for the sexual abuse. I wouldn't have had this need in me when I was younger to be a perfectionist, to always prove that I was worthy of people's acknowledgement or praise. I thought I had to be perfect. And that carried on through my married life and through my working life, and it

_____

[*] The above passage was first published in a different form in the *Toronto Star* in October 1999.

definitely led to my jumping in front of the subway. Because perfection cannot be achieved. And I was trying to be perfect and blaming myself for anything that went wrong.

After I left home I kept going to school, and I worked part-time all through high school. Then I was accepted into Ryerson Polytechnic Institute's journalism program and went there in 1980. I worked all through Ryerson and I studied a lot. I was in the top ten of my graduating class and I had two job offers. Eventually, I became a public relations officer for the Ministry of Skills Development. Six months after I got that job I jumped in front of the subway.

What led up to that? I got married to a journalist from Cambridge, Ontario, who was working at a radio station there. We'd known each other for three years in what had been a long-distance relationship. So he moved to Toronto. But the intimacy of living with a man, even though I loved him dearly, brought up all the issues from my past, about the trauma of being abused. And then the winter came on. And I hadn't realized it when I lived alone, but every winter I got depressed.

I saw a psychiatrist once a week who put me on an antidepressant, and also suggested Valium when I couldn't sleep. But he didn't talk to me. I thought: "I'm going to be like this for the rest of my life. Things are never going to get any better. If this is going to be my life, that's it. I don't want to have it."

In a way it was impulsive and in a way not. I had been practising going up to the end of the platform at the subway station and trying to walk off when I saw the train coming. And I'd been too frightened to do it. But this day at work, I had had a miserable morning; I just knew I was going to do it. I packed up my desk at work to make sure everything was in the outbox and other people could handle what was left. I put on my coat, took enough ID with me so that they would be able to identify who I was, and walked down to the subway, down to the end of the platform.

I was lucky I wasn't killed. There was a physiotherapist on the platform who, I found out later, told the emergency guys how to lift me so they wouldn't sever my spine. I spent five weeks in ICU having machines breathe for me, feed me, pee for me, everything. And they wanted to switch the machines off because they thought I wasn't going to come back to life. But my dad convinced them to keep it on for another four days, and I did come back.

When I was released, I went back to work as a clerk for the same people I'd worked for previously. It wasn't as responsible a position, but I was grateful to have anything to go back to. Unfortunately, it hadn't been explained to me what a head injury meant. It meant a lot of small deficits. I don't think as fast as I used to, so I couldn't return to journalism or public relations. My body is very different. I have a lot of pain when I'm moving quickly. I can't drive any more. I can't run. If I get fatigued everything starts to shut down; my thinking ability, my reasoning ability, my organizational ability, and my memory all go. So it really has meant the end of my career and the loss of my regular work skills, too.

I also lost my husband over it. I'm easily fatigued and I'm also quick to anger. I don't know the terminology for it, but because of this brain damage I have, I've lost the ability to foresee consequences. So sometimes when my husband and I would have disagreements, my lack of restraint would turn it into a humungous fight. We went to counselling, but basically I lost my first marriage because of that. So I'd lost my career, lost my marriage.

I wound up living on welfare. It was hard at first. It was very difficult, not being able to just run out to the corner store and buy what I needed and wanted. Not being able to go to a movie. Not being able to buy a book if I wanted, because I'm a voracious reader. Having to decide, "Okay, can I shave forty dollars off the grocery bill and buy the track pants I need?" And that gets wearying. Really wearying.

Today, I live on the Ontario Disability Support Program. They pay my rent, which is $139 a month, because it's subsidized, and then I get $516 for basic needs a month. So it's about $7,800 a year. I can find places for alternative support: I go to church lunches, I know these clothing depots where you can get things for twenty-five cents. And occasionally I can ask my dad for a bit of money. Any extra money that I do get, I save for my kids – the two boys from my first marriage –

because I see them every Saturday. I'll take them to a movie. The only movies I've seen in the last decade are kids' movies!

I have no money for entertainment – none. Again, I've found alternative things. I go to the library to read the newspaper every day. I'm a member of an art gallery called Show Gallery; I paint, and I've had a few art shows there. I know every park in Toronto, *every* park, because I've gone to visit each one.

There are good things, too, about poverty. It forces you to be creative. I ignored my artistic side totally while I was working, while I was so-called "sane." And when I became insane suddenly it was okay to paint and draw. So I started an art program for other lunatics called Hyperart.

Being a concerned volunteer has become, for me, the replacement for work. I've taken a year off from volunteer work now, but when I was active in the political psychiatric-survivor milieu, I was much in demand. If I see an injustice, it's like, "Over my dead body you're going to get away with that."

So I'm happy with my little life. I get the luxury to just be involved in things that mean something to my heart. And to really understand that the people who are walking around in crappy clothes, with their jaws hanging down making funny twitches and everything, those people aren't loonies to make fun of or to pity, they're real people. And they've all got real stories. And a lot of them have the kindest souls and the kindest hearts of anybody I've ever met. And I really enjoy advocating for people like that.

Also, having kids has made me a lot happier. It's just such a joy. And I know I'd never want to do anything to myself now, because I would not want to leave them this legacy, for them to lose a mother they love.

So I go to physio twice a week. I do a lot of walking, to make sure I get a lot of natural sunlight. I exercise. I take lithium pills three times a day to stabilize my mood. I take an antidepressant. And I see my GP every two weeks. February, the month I jumped, is the hardest month of the year for me. It was always kind of a dread thing for me – I would think all of these horrible things about February. But my psychotherapist is really good at encouraging you to do positive things. And I was talking to her about this one year, the anniversary of the jump was coming up, and she said, "Well, make it a celebration." And *bing*, like a light going on, I thought, *Make it a celebration!*

So every year I have an anniversary party with myself, sort of celebrating the fact that, "Yes, here I am!" On that day I think about all the people that I've met in the last decade, or know about, who didn't make it. But I also think about the positive stuff: the fact that I'm still here, there must be a reason. Whereas I used to think that I was no good, that I was unloved, that I must be a horrible person for all of that abuse to have happened to me, now I think, "Hey, I must be a really okay person to have been brought back from death. Because here I am!"

Sue Goodwin hopes to start a holistic mental health and addiction centre, offering advocacy, alternative treatments, and solace to the psychiatric survivor community.

ON RECOVERY: A university student from Halifax named Andrew Oland explains what it's like trying to navigate his way towards recovery from an illness like schizophrenia.

"Struggling to find your way to decent health and peace of mind while having a mental illness is like being in a massive building, with no lights and the windows bricked up, trying to find your way out in total darkness. You can only go ahead carefully, wave your arms around in front of you, and try to figure out where there's a wall and where there's a way. Sometimes you'll walk or crawl face first into a wall. Or you'll end up walking off the edge of a stairway thinking you're in the middle of a hallway. And it'll hurt, sometimes a lot, and you'll be afraid to move for a while because of it, and maybe question whether you'll ever escape or whether it'd be easier to just stay put. And sometimes you'll end up touching a door handle, joyously twisting it and flinging the door open, rushing through — and finding you're in a closet. You may not be able to get out as fast as you want to, but it's a whole lot better than the odds if you just sit on your butt and pray to be rescued. You have to do the legwork."

CHAPTER 3 WHERE THE HEART IS

◠◠◠

Home is where the heart is.

And virtually every home will be touched in some way by mental disorder.

We might not talk much about it in public, but a member of nearly every family will, at some point, experience a form of mental ill-health serious enough to impair other aspects of living. In fact, a public education campaign in Britain has been called "Every Family."

Of course, the person most directly affected is the individual with the disorder. But the impact on other family members can be monumental, and there's really no way of predicting how things will unfold.

Some families have discovered that surviving a mental disorder alongside a loved one has only strengthened their bonds; others have learned that severe and chronic illness can push relationships past their breaking point. Recent research has even suggested that depression, for example, can be "contagious," sometimes spreading to others living under that shared cloud.

When *The Last Taboo* was published in 2001, we promoted the book with a number of media interviews. At every venue, once the cameras or microphones had been turned off, the notebooks closed, someone inevitably came forward and tugged at our sleeves, whispered in our ears.

Invariably, they either had experienced a mental disorder – or had a family member who had struggled. Some of these people were very well-known media figures – proving yet again that neither money nor status "insulates" a person from mental disorder.

The following stories come from family members united by a common bond, one that perhaps even you share. They've all seen mental illness hit home.

SCOTT THOMPSON
A Brother's Story

It's something of a miracle that comedian Scott Thompson and his four brothers survived childhood intact. More specifically, that any of them withstood the crucible of the family basement in Brampton, Ontario.

"The whole family are fighters. We're very physical," Thompson says. "With five boys, all you do is hit each other. That's all we ever did. Still to this day people find me a little much . . . because we yelled all the time. And if the person wasn't listening to you, you punched them so that they'd listen to you yell, '*You're not listening to me!*' It was so normal."

As a starring member of the hit comedy troupe The Kids in the Hall, Thompson would put his childhood experiences to good use. Each week on CBC television – and now in syndication on The Comedy Network – he and the Kids parodied the chaos that brims just beneath the surface of suburban middle-class life. Often, Thompson played, in full housewife regalia, the role of the eternally patient mother.

The Kid in the Hall, however, started out as a boy in that basement. And in that wild kingdom affectionately known as "the *wreck* room," Thompson says, "There were no rules." There, young Scott gave one of his first successful performances.

Older brother Rand was babysitting Scott and younger brother Dean. "We were fighting," Scott recalls. "I was picking on the two of them. Then they picked on me. And they tried to strangle me, and I pretended I'd actually died. I kept it up. I gasped and I went through all these convulsions."

There is nothing quite so infectious as Scott Thompson, professional comedian, getting right into a good story. He gags and sputters, wheezes and contorts. His face appears a light shade of blue. When he's satisfied his guests are suitably amused, he presses ahead, explaining how his brothers kicked him, with increasing force, to prove he wasn't *really* dead. "I didn't say boo. I thought, 'I'm playing this all the way.'" (It's a trait for which he would later become famous.)

"All of a sudden I remember Dean going 'Oh, my God – WE KILLED HIM!' And then it was like, '*You* did it.' 'No, *you* did it!' . . . They were already figuring out how to make it look like it wasn't murder."

Another round of laughter. A perfectly timed pause. Then Thompson narrows his eyes to slits. "They became the Menendez brothers *immediately*."

Well, not quite. Today, brother Rand is a banking executive. Scott, on the day we meet him, has just returned from a New York appearance on a celebrity game show and is about to leave on a two-month Kids in the Hall reunion tour across North America. Fourth-in-line brother, Craig, is a professional engineer and successful Web designer, and baby brother Derek is trying his own hand at standup comedy on the Toronto nightclub circuit. "My family's very ambitious," Scott says. "Really competitive."

Dean's life, however, followed a different path. The middle child, he was "incredibly easygoing" and not remotely competitive. "Dean was actually the most normal of anyone in the family," Scott says. "He was like a classic boy: good-looking, blond, always laughed, lots of fun, really athletic. . . . All the girls loved him. He was built like a god."

Born just one year apart, Dean and Scott grew up with a special bond, playing together every day and sharing a room each night. "We were *always* together," he says. "We were thought of as kind of twins." Or if not twins, then mirror images; a fraternal yin and yang. "We were very opposite. We were very much one person. You know, one covers one side and the other covers the other."

Their parents concur: one son was the thinker, the other was the athlete. "Scott read at a very early age," mother Barbara says. "He always had his nose in a book."

Dean, meanwhile, was the high school quarterback, the teenage ski instructor, and the gifted hockey player. His almost-twin looked on with envy at Dean's God-given athletic grace. "He had muscles when he was *three*," Scott says, rolling his eyes. "When we played sports together, he just won everything, and I would always be left bleeding and gasping and covered in mud."

The high school graduation photos in the Thompson family home seem to confirm those early archetypes. There's Dean, handsome in a rugged, broad-shouldered kind of way, offering the slightest of smiles. And there's Scott, with the same shaggy blond haircut, but also with thick eyeglasses and wide grin. He looks smaller, nerdier.

The family photos – dozens of them – cover the panelled walls of the Thompsons' den. And on a corner bookshelf, alongside the photo of Scott in one of his best-loved roles – Queen Elizabeth, waving with gloved hand – sit four of his Gemini Awards. "We keep them here," father Philip explains, almost embarrassed, "because otherwise they'd just get lost."

Philip Thompson is tall and dignified, and speaks with a certain thoughtful economy. Barbara, slim and quick-moving, has thick curly hair and a warm smile reminiscent of those mother characters Scott sometimes plays on TV. "Yes," says Philip, chuckling, "he plays his mother quite well." Together, they share their memories, sitting side by side in the spotless living room adjoining the den. It's a more formal space in which tea and Peek Freans are graciously served. (One suspects the Thompson boys didn't spend much time in here.)

"I thought Scott would be a lawyer," says Philip.

Barbara nods in agreement. "Always arguing."

Dean had a gentler personality. "He was the most caring of the boys," Barbara remembers.

Scott remembers too. His younger brother, he says with a sigh, "was like me but new and improved. Bigger, stronger, faster." With another well-timed pause, he adds: "*Straighter*."

Thompson, who is openly gay, will deliver fast and funny jokes almost all evening long. It's his trademark. But he will also speak with tremendous warmth and honesty about his closest brother, and about what went wrong.

At eighteen, Scott spent a year in the Philippines as part of a Canada World Youth program. It was his first trip away from home, and his parents were soon sending him anguished letters: Dean had quit school, was drinking and behaving not at all like himself. From the other side of the world, Scott laughed all this off as mere rebellion – the good boy finally deciding to try being bad. "If only my parents knew what *I'd* been doing," he remembers thinking.

When Scott returned home to Brampton, the entire family was there to welcome him at the front door. Everyone but Dean. "I thought, 'Well, why didn't he come down to see me?' And then I saw him. He came into the foyer, and he said, 'Hey, how're you doing?' And I looked at him, and inside I went, 'What happened? Who is that?'" Thompson pauses. "It was in the eyes. . . . It wasn't him. And honestly, it never was again. That was it. That was really the end. It took, like, fifteen years for it to really end, but I guess the disease had descended that year."

The disease was schizophrenia, which would take many years to be diagnosed. For most of those years, the Thompsons were struggling to understand what was wrong.

"I would never have thought it would have anything to do with a brain disease," says Barbara, shaking her head.

"We really didn't know," adds Philip.

Scott was equally confused. "I was convinced he was faking. I never thought of it as crazy, because it wasn't what I thought crazy was."

If anything, Scott was the son with the crazy persona. "I was incredibly volatile as a kid. I went off on wild flights of fancy. I'd come home and say, 'I met a raccoon that talked to me.' And Dean would come home and say, 'I just played tennis all afternoon.' I mean, really. You're not going to say, 'Look at the blond good-looking athlete: He's the one that's going to go nuts.'"

Barbara concurs, recalling with fondness that Scott was always "into mischief. He was always living on the edge. We were rescuing him most of the time."

For years, everyone knew *something* was happening to Dean, but no one knew quite what. He was hanging around the house, writing poetry – journal after journal full of it. And reading fervently, especially such "heavy" writers as Nietzsche and Schopenhauer.

"I'd say to my mother, 'He's *fine*. He's just reading the wrong books!'" Scott says. "I'd say, 'Don't let him read Nietzsche.' . . . I really was convinced that he wasn't ready for it, and that it had warped him. Isn't that naive? But that's what I thought."

With time, Scott became convinced his brother was trying to copy him – a new take on the sibling rivalry that had always existed between them. "He started taking on qualities that were *my* qualities, like being unpredictable and reading very difficult books and talking crazy. And that's what *I* do. That's *my* job. I just kept thinking, 'You're muscling in on my territory.' . . . I have to be honest – I was not at all sympathetic. *At all.*"

Dean spent his early twenties moving back and forth from the house in Brampton to a series of apartments in downtown Toronto. He started university, then dropped out. He took jobs, but couldn't keep them. "I'd get him jobs in construction," says Philip, a civil engineer, "and he'd work for a while and then all of a sudden he just wouldn't show up."

Scott's career, meanwhile, was taking off. He was on national television every week as perhaps the wackiest of the five wacky Kids. Dean would call sometimes after a show had aired, convinced that Scott was speaking to him through the television. "There was a lot of that. 'What were you saying to me in that courtroom scene?' 'Dean, *nothing*.' And I didn't have a lot of patience." Scott leans back in his chair. "I'm not proud. I can't pretend that I was like a big hero. I was not at all."

Then one day in 1984, everything changed again. Dean was hit by a car as he was crossing a downtown street on his bicycle. So severe were his injuries that when Scott first saw him lying in a hospital bed, he fainted.

For twelve days, Dean lay in a coma. Doctors said he wouldn't live, but he did. Then they said he'd never walk or talk again. But he did. Dean spent a full year in hospital, several more in physical therapy.

"He had to learn *everything* all over again," Scott says.

"They actually used him at the hospital as an example of how determination can bring you back," his father says with pride.

During the long, painful recovery process, Scott says, the family "conveniently forgot" about the strange behaviour of the years before. "But, lo and behold, as he got better, the craziness came back. You can't imagine what that must be like. Schizophrenia *and* brain damage? I honestly think my brother would have been able to live with one or the other. But not two."

Schizophrenia. Dean had still not been diagnosed with it, but by now, the family had seen enough, heard enough, gathered enough information to suspect it applied. The telltale symptoms were all there: delusions, paranoia, social withdrawal. He'd drink too much, get into minor scrapes with the law. For more than ten years, he lived like this. And the illness took an enormous toll on everyone. Barbara and Philip could not convince their son to see a doctor. Barbara began to fear he'd wind up on the streets, lost to everyone. It consumed a lot of their time and energy. And although the other four boys were no longer living at home, they noticed.

"Everyone got jealous of the time," Scott admits. "Especially after the accident, all attention went to him. The whole family revolved around Dean . . . what to do, how to get help, where to go. It went on for a long time."

Scott and Dean's relationship deteriorated further. Dean, having taken up religion, proclaimed Scott a sinner because he was gay. (Scott had been one of the first Canadian performers to acknowledge – even flaunt – this fact; one of his best-known characters is the lisping, cravat-wearing lounge queen, Buddy Cole.) And Dean would often call to ask for money.

"We'd had some really bad fights the last couple of years, where I didn't want to talk to him any more. And I told him that." Scott hesitates before continuing. "I was embarrassed, honestly. I'm not proud of that, but I was. When he'd come to visit me at the office, I was embarrassed. I'd see him on the street, I was embarrassed. And you shouldn't be embarrassed. Especially a person in my position. I really should have understood more."

The next big turning point came in 1993, when Dean spent a night in jail. He'd been following a young woman, and as a condition of his release, he agreed to psychiatric assessment. Within a few months, schizophrenia was diagnosed, and for the first time Dean started taking medication. He was, by now, thirty-five years old.

The medication's side effects were troubling. Worst of all, for the former athlete, was the dramatic weight gain. But as he had after the accident, Dean persevered. And fairly quickly, something remarkable happened. The son and brother who'd been hijacked for more than a decade returned.

"We all said we had the old Dean back again," says his father. "He was the Dean that we knew many, many years before."

"I would connect with him again," says Scott, who had moved to Los Angeles after the *The Kids in the Hall* ended, and had by now just begun work on another hit comedy, *The Larry Sanders Show*. "He said sorry for certain things he'd done. And a week before he died, he told me that he loved me. That haunts me, because I know he was saying goodbye." It takes a while before Scott can continue. "I think what was sad was that it was when he was getting better."

The weekend before his death, Dean returned home to his parents' house. He played golf with his dad. "That was the best weekend we ever had," Philip recalls. "He hadn't played golf for years and years and years – and he could hit that ball like nothing. We had a great time. I always remember that. I thought then that things were really beginning to turn around."

The following Thursday, Barbara made her nightly phone call to Dean's apartment. She was looking forward to seeing him again on Saturday. "And this different voice answered, and I said, 'Oh, excuse me, I've got the wrong number.'" Barbara identified herself as Dean's mother. "And this gentleman said, 'No, you haven't called the wrong number.'"

Barbara Thompson looks away. "I don't really remember . . ."

"And then I talked to him," Philip gently interjects, referring to the police officer.

That night, in L.A., Scott heard the news from his brother Rand. "I'd told Dean I'd call him Thursday," Scott says. "And I didn't call him." He's tearful now, but he finishes his thought. "I know that's not the reason. But suicide's weird."

As always with suicide, the Thompsons have tried to understand that most tormenting of questions: Why did he do it? There had been no real warning signs. But Scott, Barbara, and Philip Thompson all agree that the medication, although it eased Dean's symptoms, had given him a renewed ability to assess where his life was going.

"The medication allowed him to see his life. But what he saw, he *didn't like*," says Scott. "I think he looked at himself, and for the first time he went, 'I'm thirty-five, I can't hold down a job . . .'"

Dean had been living alone, and had recently started working at an unskilled job in a hospital. "Being the competitive person he was," says Barbara, "he didn't like getting a job washing dishes. He still had his pride."

"He realized he had no friends," adds Philip, "that they had progressed and had jobs and families."

The family, as families do, held fast together for Dean's funeral. Every member of the Kids in the Hall attended, and that meant a lot. And then, slowly, the Thompsons began the work of putting their lives back together.

Seven years later, Barbara still takes comfort in the words of Dean's doctor. "He said, 'Remember, Mrs. Thompson, Dean didn't take his life – schizophrenia took his life.'"

Philip has found meaning in volunteer work with the Schizophrenia Society; he gives speeches at schools, does everything he can to eliminate the stigma. Both parents take solace in their religious faith, their friends and family. "I have to be strong," Barbara says, "for the others. Dean would want me to be."

"My parents have made quite a journey," says Scott. "They raised five boys: they have two gay sons, they had a son with schizophrenia who committed suicide. It hasn't worked out the way they expected. . . . These are people in their seventies. They know by what they've been through that you just can't control certain things. You don't choose to be gay, you don't choose to be mentally ill, you don't choose your colour or your language. That's just the way it is."

After the funeral, before he flew back to L.A., Scott paid a visit to Dean's apartment building, to the place "where his soul had left the earth." For a moment, there was an eerie double-take as the building superintendent mistook Scott for Dean. Then the man handed something to Scott. It was a pair of eyeglasses, covered in blood, found near where he died. They were Dean's.

Scott took the glasses with him to Los Angeles, carrying them everywhere. "After he died, my life was not very together for a few years. And for me it was all about loss. Just loss, loss, loss. My brother, my troupe, leaving the country, my boyfriend. I just felt like I'd lost everything." For a long time, he was, if not clinically depressed, then chronically unhappy, and his life spun out of control. "I gave up, in some ways. I was just really angry. And my health wasn't good.

"I felt terrible guilt. I think that's why you make things not work out, so that you can say to the other person, 'See? Things are bad for me too.' You just decide, I'm going to screw up my life too so that they'll feel better – which is so stupid. That's what I think I did."

Scott's health deteriorated to the point that painful welts broke out on his ankles and legs. "Bull's eyes and lashes, as if I'd been whipped." In three different hospitals, the doctors were baffled. Then finally, after months of agony, Scott read a book by Deepak Chopra. "And he said, 'Listen to your body.' He said that if it [pain] comes from your legs, your body's saying to you, 'Stop moving.'"

Thompson had been on the road for months, carrying the guilt and anger with him. He took the advice. "Since then," he says, "I won't carry it with me. I won't carry the anger. Obviously, I still have the grief. That never leaves you. That's just the modern world thinking there's such a thing as closure, which is just nonsense."

Last year, Thompson left L.A. and moved back home to Toronto. Today, as he pads around his tidy galley kitchen in thick sweat socks, a plain T-shirt and cargo pants, he looks in excellent physical shape. His chest and biceps are toned in a way Dean's perhaps once were. He's been eating healthily, working out. At his parents' request, and because the myths and misconceptions infuriate him, he's also started speaking out about schizophrenia. Giving speeches and occasional interviews.

Thompson remains extremely close with his parents and three surviving brothers. And, in his own way, with Dean, too. "Ever since he died, he's visited me," Scott says. "He watches over me."

He pauses one last time. Then quickly, he lifts the left sleeve of his T-shirt and peels off a square nicotine patch to reveal something beneath.

"See? This is him."

And there, on the back of his arm, is a simple tattoo about the size of your middle three fingers. It's a pair of eyeglasses. And in one lens a bright sun breaks through a tuft of cloud. "I had them tattooed on me so that he can watch my back," Scott says with a big smile. "And he does."

Gently, he rolls the sleeve back down over his arm.

SCHIZOPHRENIA AND SUICIDE

▶ One in every hundred people will develop schizophrenia in their lifetime.

▶ Three hundred thousand Canadians aged sixteen to thirty have been diagnosed with schizophrenia (Canadian Coordinating Office for Health Technology Assessment, 1998).

▶ The average time between onset of symptoms and first effective treatment is one to two years, but can be much longer.

▶ Males and females are equally likely to be diagnosed with schizophrenia. But males tend to have an earlier age of onset, in the teens or early twenties for men, and in the twenties or early thirties for women.

▶ Nearly 80 per cent of people with schizophrenia experience a major depressive episode at some point in their lives.

▶ Approximately four out of every ten people with a diagnosis of schizophrenia attempts suicide.

▶ Approximately one in ten people diagnosed with schizophrenia die of suicide, making it the leading cause of premature death for people with schizophrenia.

▶ "Suicide in this population is rarely attributable to florid psychotic symptoms (hallucinations, delusions); it is more likely to occur in periods of remission or improved functioning" (Health Canada, *Suicide in Canada*, 1994). The report also notes that depression and hopelessness are important factors in suicide by people with schizophrenia.

HOW SIBLINGS ARE AFFECTED

Tom Ko has worked with 160 families in his job as therapy supervisor at the Calgary Early Psychosis Treatment and Prevention Program. Many — but not all — of his clients are young enough to be living at home with parents and siblings. Ko, who has a master's degree in social work, encourages the whole family to attend psychoeducation sessions with him. "Not all siblings have strong emotional reactions to the illness," says Ko, a social worker. "But all have *some* reaction to a psychotic illness in the family."

Here are some of the common emotions and issues raised by the siblings he's seen:

1. ANGER at parents ("Why don't they take control and fix this?") and at the unwell sibling ("Why doesn't he just get better?"). "They get angry a lot because things have changed," Ko says. "They want their brother or sister back."

2. GRIEF AND SADNESS: "Because the family isn't the same, and they can sense that." Ko says that children go through a grieving process just as parents do. "When things change and everything's up in the air, they do get depressed.'"

3. FEAR that they'll become mentally ill. "Not the seven-year-old but the fourteen-year-old says, 'Will I get it?' And we are always upfront." (Research shows that if you have a first-degree relative with schizophrenia, you in turn have a 10-per-cent chance of winding up with the disorder; this compares to a 1-per-cent chance for someone with no diagnosed relatives.)

4. GUILT that they contributed to their sibling's disorder, or made it worse. For example, two brothers may have been fighting just before one is diagnosed (which is not uncommon because the sibling relationship changes with the onset of symptoms). "We try to tell them, 'You didn't know; of course you got into fights; everybody does, but it didn't cause the illness.'"

5. LOSS OF NORMAL FAMILY RELATIONSHIPS: When parents are tied up with hospitals and meds and caring for their unwell child, says Ko, "It's easy to forget there are other kids involved. . . . Often they [the siblings] will say 'we used to have family dinners together, do this and that together.' We try to get them back to those family routines so that everything goes back to normal as much as possible."

6. CONFUSION because they know something is wrong but no one is explaining what or why. "They find it very difficult to understand sometimes. They can tell their brother or sister is different, they can tell their family is different, and they wonder. But it just becomes a family secret that no one talks about. They want to know what's going on."

EUFEMIA F.
A Daughter's Story

I was fourteen years old when I found out my mother had been diagnosed with paranoid schizophrenia. That was almost twenty years ago. Thirteen years ago, I left home, and ever since I have had this recurring dream which is technically more of a nightmare. The dream begins with me visiting my parents and realizing they have had another baby. It ends with me trying to kidnap the baby, to save it from suffering the same childhood I had, filled with confusion, pain, and misunderstanding. I always wake up in a panic.

My parents were introduced to each other by my grandparents in Bonefro, Italy. My father was thirty and my mother nineteen at the time of their wedding. I found out by accident it was an arranged marriage. I was sixteen, speculating on how they spent their Valentine's days while courting, when my mother informed me there was no courtship at all. Having been raised in Canada, I had no concept of the lack of choices they endured. I was shocked and horrified. I was also relieved. All my life, I felt my parents were completely incompatible; until that point, their union made no sense. They are, however, distant cousins. This is not unusual in a small village like theirs. I tell people that, aside from DNA, my parents have nothing in common, and if I researched my family tree I'd find out I was related to myself twenty-five times.

My mother's illness was discovered in a roundabout way. In 1983, she was involved in a minor car accident and fled the scene. My father and I deliberated for hours before we called the police. As immigrants, my parents avoided authority figures as much as possible. When the police arrived, they interviewed each of us, and my father admitted, without much prompting, that my mother was difficult to live with on a daily basis. After a few questions directed to her were answered by laughter, an officer suggested my mother would probably need professional help. I remember thinking: Aha, so *we're* not crazy, *she* is.

Everything moved rapidly after that. Our family doctor was able to get my mother an appointment with an Italian-speaking psychiatrist, a major feat considering the two-month waiting list. The diagnosis was the light at the end of the tunnel of darkness and misunderstanding; years of intolerable family arguments were given an explanation. I thought a diagnosis was an explanation and that an explanation equalled a cure.

In her office, our family doctor tried to explain schizophrenia to me. She asked if I knew what it meant. I asked, Does this mean she thinks she's Napoleon one day and Christopher Columbus the next? My teenaged idea of mental illness was drawn from Bugs Bunny acting funny and a few bad movies-of-the-week.

The doctor replied, "No, what it means is, she can't hate you, but she also can't love you."

I had spent a lot of time in this particular doctor's office, crying, pouring out the details of abuse and neglect I felt proved my mother hated me. I'd spent a lot of time wondering what I could do differently to avoid the confrontations. It never worked; the rules were always changing. I would accidentally break a dish while cleaning and fear for the beating that would follow, only to find the incident shrugged off. As a picky eater, I rarely finished what was put in front of me. This was tolerated until, on a whim, I would be forced to eat everything, even if it made me gag or vomit. I never knew when the violence would erupt or what would be the cause.

So I left the office that day thinking this doctor doesn't know anything. I knew my mother hated me. She had said so. She had threatened my life on numerous occasions. And on more than one occasion, she had left me bleeding or limping, or both. Once, a few years earlier, she had bitten down hard on my hand and broken through the skin. By the time I arrived at school, I was inconsolable and incomprehensible. My homeroom teacher worried there was a rabid dog in the neighbourhood and couldn't believe his ears when I finally calmed down enough to talk clearly. Social workers were called in to interview my father and me separately. My father was incredibly ashamed and insisted the problem was under control.

My father couldn't cope with the physical abuse. To him it was absolutely unheard of that you would treat anyone, let alone your children, in this manner. He begged me not to talk to anyone. He told my teacher and my principal we would be going to Italy to solve this problem. That summer, when I was eleven, we did go to Italy, where my father found a psychiatrist to treat my mother. She was heavily medicated for a brief period, and everyone hoped the troubled times were over. I found out years later that this was actually the first time she'd been diagnosed, but afterwards my father, not fully comprehending the situation, had assumed she was cured.

For reasons I didn't understand, I was doing extremely well academically around this time. I was fortunate that many of my teachers pushed me to excel and gave me opportunities that distracted me from the horrors at home. I was Mary in the Christmas pageant. I made a speech before our school trustees. I was involved in the school play. At one point I was even enrolled in a program for kids with problematic backgrounds, and we spent some class time working at a daycare centre near the school. I remember being very busy and happy to be out of the house. While the signs of abuse were visible in gym class, the fact that I was doing well academically seemed to comfort everyone, including myself.

For years, my mother's illness was kept a secret, even in our extended family. It's extremely difficult to hide *any* illness when you attend weddings twice a year with more than 400 guests. It's also difficult in a tight-knit immigrant community. Gradually, it became obvious to everyone that there was something wrong. And slowly but steadily, we were abandoned to our fate: three miserable shipwreck survivors lost at sea. All my life I had heard Italians saying Canadians had no sense of family. Yet in response to my mother's illness, my own Italian relatives said, "It's not our problem" or "She's not our blood relative."

For a while my parents went to the psychiatrist together, until he told my father he could do nothing for my mother if she wouldn't take her medicine. My mother rejected all medicine in the belief that we were trying to kill her.

I chose to deal with the crisis by finding every book I could read on the subject. I didn't find much that helped; there wasn't anything that described my mother or my relationship with her. I read *I Never Promised You a Rose Garden*. I tried to read R. D. Laing and Thomas Szasz, and started thinking maybe my mother was just a misunderstood genius.

My other coping method was to tell everyone everything. I was tired of the secret and hoped to find someone who could understand. I had read the statistic: one in a hundred people suffered from schizophrenia. I did the math and thought there must be quite a few relatives. But it wasn't a subject people discussed.

Shortly after I left home at nineteen and moved to the West Coast, my father collapsed on the job, emotionally, mentally, and physically drained. It happened two weeks before Easter, when I was scheduled to come home for a visit. He had been hallucinating about Jesus before he'd collapsed; he thought somehow he had offended Christ. Diagnosed with diabetes, he was briefly sent to a psychiatric ward because of the hallucinations. No one called to tell me.

The first thing I noticed when I got home was my father's jitteriness. He wouldn't sit still. He paced. He couldn't sleep. He hardly ate. He told me he needed to speak with me. We waited until my mother left to buy groceries, then sat in the backyard, where, at my father's insistence, I crossed my ankles. Apparently, this would stop my mother from overhearing our conversation. My father was terrified as he explained to me that it wasn't schizophrenia holding my mother in its grip but the devil himself. She was part of a family of bad witches who could curse anyone in their path with the evil eye. She was sent to us by the devil, my father insisted, and she could cause us great harm.

She already has, I said, and this is bullshit. I felt there was no longer hope for a future of sane communications with either of them. My mother, meanwhile, was thrilled with my father's collapse, and began to say he had been the crazy one all along.

I returned to British Columbia frustrated and angry. My father was put on many different medications, and some of them clashed. He attempted suicide, and still his family kept their distance. Soon, he sought the advice of his roots – good witches who could help our family. They would remove the curse. It would take a lot of effort and some cash, of course. These women made their living as good witches and had to be compensated. A lot of time, effort, and money was spent. Items like religious medallions or prayer cards were buried in the yard or hidden in the house to counterbalance the presence of evil. At one point the local priest came by to help, blessing the house with holy water. I became disgusted and started to lose respect for my father. It was an immensely difficult time, as I had always admired his intelligence and ability to reason.

I had been living away from home for four years when I became depressed. I was twenty-three, and a university dropout. I had quit a job that made me miserable, thinking I would easily get another. When that proved impossible, my self-esteem plummeted. I went on Prozac and welfare. I lived in my pyjamas for days on end. I lost my patience and sense of humour. I spent six months crying and feeling wiped out. Then someone (thank God) offered me a job and I got back on track.

Meanwhile, my father recovered, too. We tried to make peace, but a vicious cycle emerged: an explosion from my mother, then an uneasy calm until the next reminder that she was still not well. This horror continued for years. I stayed away as much as possible, felt intensely guilty, and continued to accept my mother's abuse long-distance, on the answering machine. My only relief was that none of my room-mates ever understood her Italian dialect. For a brief period, I cut off contact, and then, because I was afraid of my father's declining health, gave in.

Recently, my father joined a support group specifically for Italian-Canadians with mentally ill relatives. Surprisingly, this came about through a phone call my mother made to the police. (Over the years they have made many visits to the house.) She called to complain that it was impossible to live with my father. Within moments of meeting my mother, the officer suggested my father needed support services and gave him a phone number. He also set up an appointment for my father.

I am so grateful for this turn of events. My father now has a group to talk with who have similar backgrounds and experiences. I had been trying for years to step down from the position of fight mediator and family counsellor. After his first few meetings I could hear the difference in my father's voice. He sounded happy. While his daily dealings with my mother are still difficult, he's not alone any more.

For many reasons I respect, my father won't abandon my mother, even when all the relatives suggest he should. My father has a great deal of empathy and doesn't want to desert my mother. He's been ridiculed for this by some of the ever-ready-to-dispense-advice members of the clan, but he is also respected for his incredible strength and his many attempts to find a solution.

I've also started attending a support group for family members. Fifteen years ago, the only support service I could find was specifically for "parents of schizophrenics." Now there is a great deal more information and awareness, although still not enough. My hope is that no one will ever have to feel alone with this painful secret again.

As for my mother, I am hopeful that things will change for the better, but I've also spent quite a bit of time on what I refer to as the "hope roller coaster." Every day is a test in patience and understanding I feel I don't always pass.

Recently, I got married. It was a beautiful day and I was so happy. My father was there, but my mother was not. I have no wish to cause her any further sadness, but the day would have been extremely stressful for her and for me if she had been present. Long before her diagnosis, I learned to make compromises and adjustments to try to make every situation less stressful. It can be exhausting.

The impact of my mother's illness has been enormous. I never take for granted a good conversation with anyone, because I know the frustration and agony of not being able to communicate with a loved one.

There are days now when we break through the barrier of the illness and my mother manages to laugh, converse, or express herself clearly. Those are the days I celebrate.

After Eufemia wrote this story for us, she was hired as a full-time researcher/writer for the British Columbia Schizophrenia Society. She is now helping to develop an educational program for family members that will be used across the country.

HOW CHILDREN ARE AFFECTED

There's a real shortage of programs aimed at helping children who have a parent with a mental disorder, but one program in B.C. has been running successfully for eight years now. Hylda Gryba is a nurse and counsellor who facilitates a group psychoeducation program for children aged eight to thirteen run by the British Columbia Schizophrenia Society. The children have a parent with schizophrenia, depression, or another mental disorder. According to Gryba, some of the common feelings and issues raised by children include:

1. OVER-RESPONSIBILITY: Children often feel it's their responsibility to make their unwell mother or father healthy again. "It's not the kid's job to make sure the parent is happy or well," Gryba says, but children often don't understand this.

2. GUILT: Children often feel they are personally to blame for a parent's ill health. "They think, 'Somehow I was not the perfect child and therefore this happened,'" Gryba says. "It's very common."

3. STIGMA: Gryba remembers one child describing how his relatives would exclude him and his mother from family gatherings and cross the street rather than say hello. "Not all of the children would relate to that," Gryba says, "but a lot of them do." Children also experience stigma in the schoolyard or playground, when other kids make comments about mental illness.

4. SHAME: This is related to stigma. Children can feel inferior or that they are somehow defective if their parent is mentally ill. "It's a family shame," Gryba explains, "being embarrassed by things that the parent does around other people. I remember one girl saying, 'I don't want people to know that she's my mom.'"

5. CONFUSION AND FEAR: Children might not understand why a parent, when unwell, is sometimes short-tempered or reacts with an angry outburst. "It's not understanding why they get blamed or why the emotionality [from a parent]." Gryba helps the child to identify problem situations, and the emotions that go with them. "What's important is that you as an individual understand how you feel and why."

Not all children, of course, will experience all of these emotions. But they all can benefit from learning the kinds of coping skills that provide ways of dealing with difficult situations or feelings.

THE NEXT GENERATION

▶ Parental mental disorder is a significant risk factor for behavioural and emotional problems as well as mental disorders (including depression, panic disorder, phobias, and alcohol dependence) in children and adolescents.

▶ The link is especially strong for depression. Twenty to 50 per cent of depressed children and adolescents have a family history of depression. Non-adult children of depressed parents are more than three times as likely as other children to experience a depression. The 1999 U.S. Surgeon General's report on mental health states, "It is not clear whether the relationship between parent and childhood depression derives from genetic factors or whether depressed parents create an environment that increases the likelihood of a mental disorder developing in their children."

▶ Parental disorder is also a risk factor for developing a mental disorder as an adult. A major Ontario health survey has found that, of several risk factors investigated, the strongest single factor for mental disorder was "evidence of mental disorders in one or both parents."

HEATHER RILEY[*]
A Wife's Story

If you want to see God laugh, tell him your plans. When I met my husband, I was certain that I was planning a life of stability. Looking back, that seems absurd.

I met Steven at the end of a volatile, passionate, painful relationship, and immediately after the suicide of a close friend. I was consciously looking for my "rock" in the midst of unexpected pain. And Steven was an exemplary rock. He was loyal, resolute, responsible, brilliant, and serious. I had no doubt that he would be a good provider and a

---

[*] Heather and Steven Riley are pseudonyms.

faithful mate. We were young, but I felt safe in my choice, and we married at twenty-four.

We had both completed graduate programs in the United States, and decided to make our lives there. Before we could blink, we were gainfully employed homeowners expecting our first child. When our daughter was born with a disability, Steven's unwavering support reassured me that I had chosen my partner wisely. He helped me manage my grief in the face of her diagnosis with remarkable composure.

Months passed, and my feelings of disappointment were slowly transformed into pride and hope. Steven, too, seemed to be looking to the future, and began to consider more lucrative professional pursuits. We decided to move back to Toronto so that I could be nearer to my family and he could explore his career interests. The move included the purchase of a beautiful new home as well as a promising job for Steven, but already I was noticing a subtle yet frightening deterioration of his mood. By the time our first child was one, I was pregnant with our second, and I was certain of the change in my husband.

It is hard to characterize those initial months of concern. The same qualities that I had so admired in Steven were now stretched to alarming extremes. Whereas his sense of responsibility had once made me feel safe, he was now consumed with our finances and expressed irrational dissatisfaction with the choices we had made. This was troubling to me, because we were financially secure, living in a beautiful home, realizing all of our hopes and dreams.

Steven seemed aloof, detached from the most critical decisions affecting our lives. I remember having to choose whether or not to undergo prenatal testing (an extremely difficult choice for me to make), and Steven seemed not to care even remotely. Months later, while I laboured on the delivery table, joyfully anticipating the arrival of our second daughter, Steven's face was full of dread. Indeed, most of his days seemed to be tempered with dread. Our battle had begun.

It was a couple more months before I forced Steven to acknowledge his mood. By then, as I now know, he was dangerously suicidal but doing his best to go through the "normal" motions of life. I was distracted by the chaos of caring for a newborn and, frankly, was terrified to admit my worst fears.

Steven was spending almost all of his time at work, and when he was home, he was angry and frustrated. Although I understood the professional pressures on him, I was sleep-deprived and emotionally depleted, and I needed my partner's support.

Most of our arguing had to do with the care of our children. While I knew Steven loved the girls, he was almost completely uninvolved with their care. The baby was extremely fussy, and I was averaging three hours of sleep each night. After six weeks of this virtually unbearable routine, I pleaded with him one afternoon to take the baby for just one hour so I could sleep. I was so rundown that my body was trembling. Steven held our crying baby for five minutes, then angrily marched upstairs, put the baby firmly down on the bed next to me, ordered me to deal with her myself, and slammed the door. Hours later, when he came to bed, I blurted out that I wanted a divorce.

Looking back, that moment was defining. After trying for so many months to ignore our worsening situation, I had uttered the ugly D-word. This helped push him to seek treatment, and the months that followed were filled with therapy, mood-altering drugs, disability leave, and frenzied attempts to restore order. Steven was diagnosed almost immediately with depression, and although it would be months before we knew how serious it was, I was extremely hopeful we were now on course for recovery. Steven, however, was skeptical, and when several medications and therapies proved ineffective, he became even more despondent.

For more than a year, I went through the motions of my life with little perspective or insight. I knew Steven was sick; I knew that I was miserable and tired. But my fantasies about our future prevailed, and I harnessed all of my energy to care for the people I loved. As a mother, I recognized my role as nurturer and comforter. I continued to shoulder almost 100 per cent of the child-rearing responsibilities; I stopped entertaining friends and family; I began working again to alleviate some of Steven's (unwarranted) concerns about money. Most of my choices were made with Steven's interests in mind first and fore-most, with the children placing a strong second.

I put all of my own needs on hold to accommodate his, since Steven was the one who was sick. At one point, Steven, in a state of utter desperation, wanted to move back to the U.S. He felt that if he returned to his old job, and to a city with a lower cost of living, his depression might improve. My instincts left me feeling dubious and sick at the prospect – our baby was just months old, I was finally feeling comfortable with the special therapies I had found for our older daughter, we had just moved into a new home, and I was relying heavily on friends and family for emotional support. However, Steven can be very convincing, especially in a state of depression. I ultimately – and un-believably, in retrospect – agreed to the move, even *with* the understanding that our marriage would likely fail; by this point, he was predicting its demise on a daily basis.

By agreeing to move, I was agreeing to leave what little security I had in my life, and I was prepared to do so, anticipating that I would soon be a single mother. In a bizarre way, it seemed to make sense; if it was going to give Steven even the slightest relief from his depression, I was glad to do it.

Steven, on the other hand, battled his depression only *outside* our family. When I pushed for marital therapy, he compared it to offering a drink to someone plummeting to death in a fiery plane crash. He said he could not save his marriage without first saving his life. While I understood this intellectually, I was heartbroken. I felt completely lost and alone.

In the three years since Steven's illness first emerged, his depression has affected my life in profound ways. Yet, when I reflect now on what has happened *beyond* trying to deal with the depression, I am always surprised. My parents divorced, I was immersed in parenting two young children (one of whom had special needs), we bought and sold three homes, I became an aunt, I returned to work, and I was still not even thirty years old. All this occurred within the context of daily visits to the hospital, heart-wrenching discussions about suicide, financial insecurity, and physical exhaustion.

I remember telling Steven that I felt as though I was disappearing. I existed only to soothe my husband and children. I knew that I had at one time been a spirited, enthusiastic, curious, and ambitious woman with varied interests and many friends. But I now felt resigned, reclusive, and very uneasy.

A turning point materialized through my new job: an opportunity to be away from Steven for a month. It was an easy decision to make. Being away from Steven, I felt free to experience my emotions without guilt or frustration. I was able to read, exercise, and enjoy my children without the impact of depression looming large. I could laugh and not feel foolish for experiencing joy. I could spend time with friends and not worry that it was causing Steven stress. I stopped walking on eggshells, and I started soothing *myself*.

When I returned, Steven was already living in a treatment facility in another city. I, with a new-found sense of equanimity, was no longer prepared to relinquish all of my needs. I was prepared to compromise; I was even prepared to bend 99 per cent of the way. I just needed to hold on to a small fraction of myself if we were to continue being married.

At the top of my list was a resolve to stay in Toronto. I was no longer prepared to make the move until we had at least one year of good marital and mental health behind us. The prospect of being divorced *and* isolated was too much to bear. Needless to say, Steven reacted badly, accusing me, in very nasty terms, of being unfair. At that moment, I knew the marriage was over. If there was no room in the marriage for my needs to be considered, then there was no room in it for me.

I had been contemplating a separation since that fateful day when my baby was just six weeks old. A year and a half later, I was convinced that it was necessary. The decision was less a function of how I felt about Steven than it was of how I felt about myself. I knew that my husband had almost no control over how he was behaving, and I actually felt very little anger toward him as a result. But I also knew that I deserved to be treated with respect and love. I shared my decision with Steven on the telephone, feeling guilty, sad, regretful, but also, for the first time in a long while, hopeful.

It has been more than a year since our separation, a year filled with practical concerns, but much emotional relief. While I miss the illusion of lifelong partnership and love, I derive great comfort in knowing that I am able to put myself first. I am no longer lost.

Steven and I speak regularly, not just for the sake of our children. I still care about him very much. I miss many aspects of him, and wish we had found our way together. But with two young daughters, and my own need for stability and support, I was simply unable to meet his very demanding emotional needs without completely neglecting my own. Steven continues to battle his demons with remarkable determination, and I am still hopeful that he will ultimately win the war.

I have asked myself whether I would want to reconcile if that happens. It is so hard to know where depression ends and personality begins. And the insecurity I have already experienced makes me terrified of a relapse.

My children are the innocent victims of this experience. I am not sure which is better for them: enduring separation from their father for the sake of relative stability and security, or living in an intact family, potentially at the expense of my well-being. I imagine I will never know the answer to that one. I do believe that I am a better mother since Steven and I separated, and that is reassuring.

Arguably the hardest lesson for me has been to discover that while mental illness is horribly stigmatized and misunderstood, the other extreme is just as dangerous. Depression is an illness, but it does not give a person licence to be mean, or insensitive, or selfish. When you love someone who is depressed, the temptation to indulge the illness is overwhelming. And while I would never suggest that we go back to an archaic "*snap out of it*" attitude, the blindness of love can be self-defeating.

Steven has missed out on so many of life's blessings because he is forever consumed with the perils of the future. I, meanwhile, have emerged from this struggle with a greater sense of peace, a greater appreciation for the many gifts in my life, a renewed gratitude for my health and the health of my children, and a better ability to live in the moment. More than anything, I have emerged with stronger convictions about the value of my own needs and feelings. Never again will I disappear, even in the face of love.

Heather Riley works as a community advocate for non-profit agencies.

IN SICKNESS AND IN HEALTH

▶ Studies suggest that stress, conflict levels, communication problems, and divorce rates are higher when one or both spouses have a mental disorder.

▶ Marriage is a protective factor against mental disorder — but only for men. That is, men who are married are less likely to develop a disorder than men who aren't, but the same association does not hold true for married women. In fact, unhappy marriages are considered a risk factor for depression in women.

▶ Depression may be particularly tough on relationships, as a review paper published in the *American Journal of Psychiatry* concludes: "A number of studies suggest that depressive illness is associated with more family distress and impairment than are other psychiatric illnesses and some medical conditions." The paper also notes that research findings suggest family members are most disturbed by the depressed person's lack of interest in social life, fatigue, feelings of hopelessness, and constant worrying.

▶ Depression may be "contagious." Spouses are at risk for becoming depressed themselves. "An estimated 40 percent of well partners of depressed people . . . are themselves so overburdened that they are candidates for professional help. Female partners are likelier than males to tilt into overload because of their multiple roles" (*When Madness Comes Home*, by Victoria Secunda).

TOM MORRIS
A Husband's Story

As the husband of a survivor, I have received kudos for "hanging in" and "being such a great guy" by well-meaning friends and family. It's tough, there's no doubt. It's the highest mountain I've ever faced. But seeing Valerie's courage as she battles for her very life year after year is a humbling experience. It's a tribute to that fuzzy concept we call the human spirit. It's a lesson for anyone who cares to listen. And this desperate battle is, amazingly, conducted by the mind against itself!

Valerie and I met in 1980 in an Irish pub in downtown Toronto, both being fans of rebel music. I was struck at once by her logic and no-nonsense approach and, because I'm a fair bit older than her, by the fact we shared just about everything in our outlooks. We married in 1985 and began building our lives just like everyone else – work, leisure, travel, planning our future, and, of course, indulging in our second shared passion, living with cats. Little did we know, our first cat, Wilis, was destined to provide an island of serenity during the many storms we would soon face.

Valerie worked in information technology, and I, as a social housing provider. We lived in downtown Toronto until 1998, when we purchased our bungalow in Whitby, Ontario, and, having lost Wilis to old age, joyfully enlarged the Morris cat population to four girls – Pearl, Cozette, Fontyne, and Molly – four islands of serenity. Without them ever having read a word about mental disorder or consulted a psychiatrist about it, we have absolutely no doubt our cats know exactly how Valerie is feeling and just what to do – whether to frolic and make her laugh, or to surround her with warm, purring bodies and give her peace.

Our journey into the world of bipolar disorder began in earnest about 1993, although now that we understand the process, many signs were there long before. It's amazing what knowledge can uncover, because as the tape is played back, what I thought was just Valerie's occasional moodiness and "strange" behaviour were in fact the opening salvos of the frontal attack soon to come.

The second half of February 1993 was to be an exciting two weeks sharing a beach house with friends in the Florida Keys. But only days into the vacation, Valerie had her first (to my knowledge, although I now doubt it) severe attack of depression. And, as many victims do, she not only suffered the attack publicly, she endured the impatience, if not downright hostility, of those whose structured lives were being disrupted. "Get over it! We've only got two weeks!" we all told her as she opted to lay in bed during those gorgeous sunny days while the rest of us did the tourist thing. "What's wrong with her?" my friends asked. I shrugged, confused and annoyed.

Val had been seeing a psychiatrist for a short time before this, but was firmly convinced he didn't understand her and was of no help. In fact, she had a plan. On our return to Toronto, and on her doctor's advice, we visited a well-known psychiatric clinic for what everyone (except Valerie) believed was to be an assessment, a second opinion. I was privately interviewed first and gave the usual uninformed responses. Valerie was next. In less than ten minutes the doctors flew into the waiting room and announced they would be admitting her. Valerie had just calmly informed them that she hadn't come to the clinic for herself. She was there for me. I would need their help, she told them, to cope in the world she would shortly be departing.

Leaving her there was the last thing I had expected. There was no effort by the doctors to describe the dangers, no time taken to outline her condition – we had not, to that point, even heard the word "depression" spoken. The debate revolved around the Mental Health Act and the scope of a doctor's authority. It was quite a scene and it took my promise to "be responsible for her" to escape the place. What now?

The next five years were, for Valerie, a maze of seeking help, rejection of the problem, acceptance of the problem, attempts at self-destruction, admissions to the seventh floor of our north Toronto hospital for short and lengthy stays, electroshock treatments, pills, pills, and more pills, the side effects of which made a cruel mockery of medications, and months away from work. To this day, our little joke as we drive past that hospital is to raise our fists in mock revolutionary salute and yell, "Free the Seventh Floor Seven!"

I'm not certain, but I think I actually first grasped the words "clinical depression," "manic depression," and "bipolar disorder" in an emergency room of that same hospital some time in 1994 as a doctor and I stood over Valerie late one horrible night. She lay in a daze, the charcoal forced into her stomach (to soak up the mix of pills and alcohol) blackening her lips and staining her hospital gown.

But from this first attempt at suicide through to others, I see the will to live. I see that spark struggling against terrible odds not to be stamped out. I see a gigantic battle going on within. If such heroism doesn't inspire, not much on this earth will.

My own process proceeded from bewilderment to frustration to gradually learning the mechanics of bipolar disorder and the infinite depths of Val's strength. From the start this was obviously going to be a race with our own ignorance. We were either going to learn all we could about the disease in a hurry, fight back with unity of purpose and armed with valid information, or lose Valerie.

In the early, undiagnosed stages, my bewilderment and frustration had stemmed from sudden mood changes in someone I loved. With no tools, no information, no clues that I might recognize, and certainly no experience to fall back on, I did what most people probably do, which was to draw other conclusions, ranging all the way from "having a bad day" to "having an affair."

This early period was in many ways the most difficult, precisely because of our ignorance of what was happening. Certainly, Valerie couldn't explain to me what she herself couldn't understand. For patients' partners it's also, I believe, the most dangerous stage, because, basing our words and actions on a complete misunderstanding of what is happening, we quickly become part of the problem and not part of the solution as we rampage about feeling upset, frightened, angry, and betrayed. As we do, we add miles to the road the patient is travelling . . . and that's my free commercial in favour of early diagnosis and a speedy understanding of the disease.

All these years, except for the worst days (which usually come just before taking Valerie into hospital for peace, recovery, and treatment lasting about a week), I go to work and try to keep a "normal" schedule. Somewhere in the mass of advice and information dumped on me, I heard that keeping a routine is important so as not to be overwhelmed. "You're not much help if you get sick over this," someone told me early on. It seemed trite at the time, because I did feel sick. But it continues to work for me and was good advice.

As well, friends, family, co-workers, and neighbours all needed to be brought up to speed. Like me, they needed a crash course on what bipolar disorder is – and isn't – and what they could do to be of help. I was lucky, and am very grateful, because everyone did what had to be done, which in most cases has meant simply understanding what is happening in our family and making allowances when necessary.

As difficult as this path has been, it was made even more so by the attitudes of some in the medical profession who completely disregarded any role by partners, friends, or family. With some psychiatrists, I had to consistently struggle to stay connected with what was happening to Valerie during her time in hospital. It seemed logical to me that an informed partner is essential in the overall recovery – after all, we spend far more time with the patient than doctors do. Yet I was often considered a nuisance for asking questions, and in one case was simply left out of the information loop as Val endured a series of electroshock treatments (treatments she regrets). There was no consultation with or explanation to either of us before this drastic procedure, and certainly none afterward. In fairness, we found other doctors – and in almost every case, nurses and crisis workers – to be understanding and caring.

In so many ways, Valerie's illness has brought us much closer than we might otherwise have been. It tests us both. How small the petty annoyances of life become as we endure this trial by fire. What a victory it is to be here, to be together, to be frustrating the beast. How we appreciate the achievements of the many people with mental disorders who have, in the past, contributed greatly to society, realizing as we do how hard they struggled, and at what cost, as they led nations, produced art and literature, excelled in science and technology.

On so many occasions, Valerie has attempted to describe to me what the torment is like; how it twists illogic into logic, how it is all-encompassing, all-pervasive. She speaks of the hopeless void, the numbness, the fear of the unknown and the known, of being fearful when you are sad because it will never end, and fearful when you're happy because it will.

How to understand all this? Oddly, I consider myself fortunate to be allowed a glimpse into this strange, terrible world. We decided long ago not only to face up to the illness but to speak about it to our friends, family, and workmates, openly and unashamedly.

It's an illness, not a weakness. It's treatable. It's demanding and frightening. It's a lifetime companion. It requires knowledge and patience to overcome. It takes strength to survive. It's misunderstood. It's widespread in its many forms and degrees. It's a part of our human condition.

What am I learning in all this? I hear the wonderful Welsh poet Dylan Thomas, himself a sufferer, in a cry of anguish urge his dying father: "Do not go gentle into that good night / Rage, rage against the dying of the light." Thomas was right. He believed, as I do, that not only are our illnesses a part of the human condition – so, too, are the struggles we wage against them.

We are sorry to report that after this story was first published, Tom Morris's wife, Valerie, died by suicide.

HOW SPOUSES ARE AFFECTED

Elva Crawford is a psychiatric nurse (recently retired) who co-led an eight-week workshop for spouses at AMI-Québec, a self-help organization in Montreal. All participants had a husband or wife with a mental disorder. "For that hour and a half each week, it was all about the spouses," Crawford says. They raised several issues and emotions that surfaced at times in their marriages, including:

▶ SADNESS AND LOSS – Crawford explains this as the feeling that "this isn't the person I married, and where can I find that person again?"

▶ **ANGER AND UNCERTAINTY** — A spouse might wonder, "When is this ever going to end?" The same feelings of anger and uncertainty may arise during recovery in anticipation of a reoccurrence.

▶ **CONTROL AND RESPONSIBILITY**, especially around treatment — For example, how much responsibility should a spouse take in ensuring their partner takes his or her medication? "At the end of the day," Crawford says, "we all know you can't control anybody except yourself."

▶ **WHO AND HOW MUCH TO TELL** — At the office, even among friends, spouses often wonder, "How much information do I give, how much do I explain?"

▶ **FINDING SUPPORT OUTSIDE THE HOME** — People were unclear where to turn for much-needed support. "Other people who have been there are maybe your best supports," says Crawford in recommending groups like AMI-Québec.

All of the above can occur in *any* intimate partnership. Crawford tries to normalize these experiences and emphasize that every relationship — with illness or not — takes work.

RONNIE AND WANDA HAWKINS
A Mother and Father's Story

The nicknames flow like guitar riffs. The Hawk. Mr. Dynamo. To John Lennon he was "Sir Ronnie," and according to that sax-playing fellow Arkansan, Bill Clinton, he is a "living legend." Bob Dylan called him "my idol," and Jerry Lee Lewis says he's "one of the greatest kings of rock and roll."

The Ronnie Hawkins story is, by now, pure lore. In 1958, he took off from rockabilly's heartland in the American South and landed in the hinterlands of Canada, where for years he tore up Toronto's Yonge Street strip with backflips and camel walks and rip-roarin' music. Along the way, he set up an informal on-stage rock school from which emerged The Band and other true homegrown talent. As one rock writer put it, "He may have missed the big time himself, but he sure helped to usher it in for others."

Hawkins himself is self-mocking, telling anyone who'll listen that he's just a southern redneck, a Geritol gypsy, a legend in his spare time. Then again, the man is known for his one-liners, his gift of the drawling gab. And these are very much on display one night on Yonge Street as the Hawk has another gig, at the former Nickelodeon, now grandiloquently called Top O' The Square. Here, where the doormen are meaty, the curtains are faded red velvet, and the dinner part of dinner-and-show is rubbery roast beef with over-boiled potatoes, Ronnie is clearly in his element. He has, as he likes to say, been singing in joints like this "since the Dead Sea was only sick."

"Thirty-two years ago we started this little room," Ronnie croons to the audience, and some of them surely remember. The crowd is an odd mix of grey-haired ladies in evening suits and hip young guys in black leather jackets. Ronnie himself stands on stage in dark shades, a tuxedo (satin piping, wide lapels) loose against his sizeable frame, and a red bandana around his neck.

One by one, he introduces his band, this latest incarnation of The Hawks, all mullet-headed and middle-aged. They've been around the block almost as many times as Ronnie has. Almost, because *no one's* been around rock and roll longer than Ronnie.

"I'll be the first one to make it to fifty years in the business," he's told us, surprised at his own longevity. "Everybody else is either dead or behind me."

"He's supposed to be semi-retired," his wife, Wanda, sighs. "But I guess he was a little bored."

For the past few months, Hawkins has been whipping his new band into shape, rehearsing in a huge barn behind his house. They are, he promises, "the most powerful band, music-wise, I've ever put together" – some statement, given his track record. He's also working on a new CD. Co-produced by David Foster (whom Hawkins once fired for putting too many chords into "Bo Diddley") and Robin Hawkins (Ronnie's son), it features such former Hawks as Levon Helm and

Robbie Robertson, as well as some newer talent from The Tragically Hip, Wide Mouth Mason, and Big Sugar. "I mixed all these different Canadians in with some of the old-timers," Ronnie tells us. "I like it. I don't know if anybody else will."

Meanwhile, at Top O' The Square, he's closing down another set. "This won us a Juno back in 1856 or '57," he deadpans, and the band starts playing "Lowdown." As he sings, he leans hard on the mike, a high-voltage grin on his broad face, silver hair still flowing down to his shoulders. After countless renditions of "Mary Lou," "Forty Days," and "Bo Diddley," he still exudes a certain raw enthusiasm. At sixty-six, he still looks like he's having fun.

Over the years, the Hawk has adeptly maintained his own image as a quintessential hard-drinkin', hard-livin' rocker. But that's only part of the picture. The other part exists quietly at Hawkstone Manor, on 200 acres overlooking a grand lake in picturesque Ontario farm country. This is where he lives with Wanda, his wife of thirty-nine years. She's a small woman with a full laugh, a black hairband in her long, straight strawberry-blond hair, and clear blue eyes that look clever. Being married to the Hawk, she quips, is like "being at Disney World on Space Mountain going backwards." Hawkins responds, as always, by saying he considers Wanda "the luckiest girl in the world."

Their sprawling eight-bedroom bungalow serves as a bed and breakfast in summer, and on this winter day houses six cars, two satellite dishes, and an animal-shelter's worth of dogs and cats, including six chihuahuas whose toe nails go *click, click, click* on the kitchen linoleum. In the living room, there's a piano that once belonged to Oscar Peterson and has since been hand-painted with three of da Vinci's angels – one for each of the Hawkins children.

Hawkins' fame and financial fortune have gone up and down over the course of his career, but the one constant in his life has been his family. Some say this is the very reason superstardom has eluded him. Married at twenty-seven, with the kids following soon after, he pretty much stopped touring; hence the years on the Yonge Street club scene, which kept him home and the cash flowing. "I made the choice," he once told the *Boston Herald*. "I had kids and I wanted to see them grow up. I didn't want to travel much."

Ronnie sent the kids to fancy private schools and hoped they'd grow up to be doctors or lawyers. But all three caught the music bug early. No doubt it was inevitable; they'd grown up with rock stars – Bob Dylan, Robbie Robertson, Jerry Lee Lewis – jamming in their home with their already larger-than-life dad.

A wall of photos in the living room is testament to this fact. Here, you'll find Ronnie at various ages and styles of dress with Johnny Cash, Dolly Parton, Kris Kristofferson. In one photo, he stands beside "Wild Willy" in the Oval Office, the recently inaugurated president grinning beneath a Hawk baseball cap; the accompanying scrawl reads *Enjoyed the visit, Bill Clinton*. Then there's the black-and-white print marking the week-long visit of John Lennon and Yoko Ono back in 1969. Lennon, in cape and cap, stands on the front step beside a straight-faced Ono; before them, the two Hawkins boys grin from deep within their snowsuits.

Today, one of those boys, Robin, is a professional guitar player; he and his sister Leah, a singer, often join their dad on stage. And what of the other boy, that beaming seven-year-old who, Wanda says, "wasn't really a Beatles fan" when John Lennon came visiting?

Ron Jr., their eldest child, was the most like his dad. He had the same solid face, thick dark hair, and playful personality – all traits going back several generations in Hawkins men. "He was a kidder and a trickster and a joker," Wanda recalls, smiling. "He was very, very clever. . . . He could do anything very quickly." And that included playing guitar. "We had guitar players living with us all the time, and they'd show him. And he was as good as they were at the same age."

Ronnie Jr. practised hard, listened hard to records hand-picked by Dad (Chuck Berry, Fats Domino), and by the age of fourteen showed real promise. "He would've been the greatest guitar player I'd ever seen," says Ron Sr. "I had him geared to put an album out picking. He was ready to go."

But one day, the protégé put away his guitar. He stopped playing, started hanging out in his room, refusing to come out. "One day I came in and Wanda said, 'Ronnie must be sick, he's not coming out of his room.' And that's how it started. He put his guitar down and hasn't touched it much ever since."

Ronnie Jr. also started fighting with his brother, showing flashes of anger they'd never seen in him before. "He started being vulgar to me, verbally abusive," Wanda says. "That was so out of context for him to do that. . . . We immediately started to look for help because this was not my typical son."

The next two years were a whirlwind of doctors, hospitals, vague answers. "We knew something wasn't right," Ronnie says, "but we were still hoping and praying." Ron Jr. was taken to the best treatment centres on the continent, but he was repeatedly misdiagnosed. At a hospital in Texas, Wanda was told it was "just adolescence" and given a prescription for tranquilizers. In Toronto, the diagnosis was behavioural problems. "They right away assumed," Wanda says, "because it was the seventies, that it had to be drugs." From there, Ron Jr. was sent to Montreal. In a treatment program for young addicts and alcoholics, he was placed in a room and surrounded by fellow teens who pointed at him, shouted, and urged him to "take control." Completely overwhelmed by the experience, he wound up in the hospital. (Wanda and Ronnie say that although their son experimented a little with marijuana, drugs were never the real problem.) While Ron Jr. was in hospital, Wanda was told her son had brain damage; doctors later phoned back to say they'd read the wrong file.

At this point, Ronnie Sr. was in rural Montana, filming the Kris Kristofferson movie *Heaven's Gate*. It was the start of a new career, Hawkins's first movie role, and he was excited about playing the part of villainous Major Woolcott. But the shooting soon fell behind schedule and the twelve-hour days were physically gruelling. Hawkins was forty-four years old and many of his scenes were on horseback. "He had this ruptured hiatus hernia and was being made to ride up and down rocky terrain with 75 pounds of clothing on," former band member B. J. Cook recalled in *The Hawk*. "By the end of the day the insides of his legs were like hamburger meat."

Meanwhile, Wanda was on the phone each day, frantically filling him in on her latest grilling by the doctors back home. "The tests that they put me through!" she says, still angry. "Quizzing me as if I was a bad mother. . . . I felt guilty, like I was a bad person. That's how they intimidated me."

Ronnie flew home twice to meet with the doctors and help Wanda. "I had to take a break to come in and see what was going on," he says. "Wanda couldn't handle it."

Finally, the family was given a diagnosis: schizophrenia.

"I couldn't even *say* it," Wanda recalls. "And of course it frightened me to death – you don't know what it is, and you don't know how bad it is or what even it meant."

Wanda's sense of humour and conviction appears to abandon her for just a moment. Her blue eyes fill with a profound sadness, a faraway look instantly recognizable to anyone who's been where she's been. "It was all frightening, I'm sure, to him," she says quietly. "I equate it as being in a nightmare, and living the nightmare, and not being able to wake up. And living it all the time. And to be awake and in a nightmare is frightening."

Ronnie Jr. spent a year living on a farm, at a mental health facility for young people. He tended the gardens, worked with the animals, and did well in the quiet, structured space. But the facility was for youths only, so when he reached adulthood, he moved back home and was for years in and out of hospital, the doctors trying countless different medications, Ronnie enduring countless side effects. "One made him lose so much weight that he looked like he was from Biafra. Another one made him so bloated that he looked like he could've burst," Wanda says. In all, they figure, Ronnie has been seen by more than 100 doctors over the years.

"At first I thought it might have been my fault," Wanda says. "What did I do when he was a baby? What didn't I do? What could I have done? What did I miss? I searched myself for all the reasons, and I felt – not guilty. I didn't feel that anything I did was not in the best interests of looking after my child. So I cleared myself of that."

"We thought of all kinds of if-onlys," Ronnie Sr. says. "Ronnie could've been about anything that he wanted. Because he was blessed with some smart genes. He could've done it all." Then he pauses, laughs, and quotes his buddy Jerry Lee Lewis. "The old rocker was crazy as a loon, but one thing he came up with, he said, 'You can't question God.' If it happens, it happens. All you can do is do the best you can."

Today, as he approaches forty, Ronnie Jr. is doing relatively well on a drug called clozapine, which Wanda had read about years ago. "I had begged them from the beginning to give him clozapine," she says, shaking her head. "But they thought it was best that they try all these other things first." Her anger is palpable; she feels a lot of years have been wasted.

Clozapine has eased the hallucinations and improved Ron Jr.'s awareness and memory. He now lives at a farm for adults and comes home for regular visits.

"But I wish for more," Wanda says. "I know he's capable of more."

"His talk is perfect, he remembers everything," Ronnie says, "But he has no ambition. He doesn't want to do anything or show emotion very much. So that's the other thing we're hoping they can find."

Ron Jr. is not comfortable speaking about himself with strangers, but his parents have both become extremely vocal about schizophrenia, doing talk shows and benefit concerts, using the Hawk's profile to raise money and awareness. "We do everything we can," he says. "We're hoping they're gonna find a cure, like everybody."

In return, they receive letters and e-mail from across the country, from young families just beginning to cope with schizophrenia. Wanda is encouraged by the stories; many young people are now responding well to early treatment. But there's personal sadness there, too. "I feel Ronnie missed out. He was born too early, when they didn't have the knowledge. And he has to suffer because of it."

Like most parents, Wanda has a dream for her son, a vision of the future that has nothing to do with guitars or rock and roll. "My hope," she says, "is that I will be alive to see him better. For him to wake up and say to me, 'You won't *believe* this nightmare I was in.'"

Wanda smiles, seeing it before her. "That's what I'm hoping for. I feel my whole life would be worth living for, for that. And that would be my reward."

Ronnie Hawkins' new CD, Still Cruisin', *was released in April 2002 by his own Hawk Records label.*

DOPE, DRUGS, AND PSYCHOSIS

Psychotic disorders often start in the teen years — precisely the time when many young people are experimenting with marijuana, booze, and other so-called "soft drugs." Is this coincidental or not? And if not, then the old chicken-and-egg question arises. Do some people take drugs and alcohol to "self-medicate" for symptoms not yet diagnosed? Or does substance use trigger a psychotic illness? The answer is probably a little of both.

Substance use is "a very large risk factor," says Dr. Ashok Malla, program director at the Prevention and Early Intervention for Psychoses Program (PEPP) in London, Ontario. "And it very likely is a trigger. It certainly is a trigger for relapses." (Some — but not all — studies have found that substance use is associated with higher rates of relapse and hospitalization.)

Research also suggests that substance abuse is more likely to be a problem for people with schizophrenia if they are younger, male, and have depressive symptoms. "If you do have either a propensity towards illness or you already have the symptoms, it may actually feel that it's helping, it's calming you down. And yet, it actually does make things much worse," Dr. Malla says.

Like so much about mental disorder, there are still plenty of unknowns.

RECENT RESEARCH ON SCHIZOPHRENIA

In the 1950s and 60s, and into the 70s, many psychiatrists believed that "schizophrenogenic mothers" — cold, distant, and unaffectionate — were at the root of schizophrenia. While that idea has now been abandoned, the true causes are still not known. Genetic research continues apace, but there is general consensus that genes alone do not cause schizophrenia; rather, they create a genetic *vulnerability* that combines with other unknown factors to create the disorder. As Daniel Weinberger, a senior researcher at the National Institute of Mental Health in the United States has noted, "It is very clear that genes confer risk but not fate. There has to be some second hit, something else that happens."

Some of those other factors — the "second hits" — most recently studied include:

▶ OLDER FATHERS: In a paper published in 2001, researchers in Israel reported that a father's age was "a strong and significant predictor of the schizophrenia diagnoses." Specifically, the older the father, the greater the incidence of schizophrenia among his children. "These findings support the hypothesis that schizophrenia may be associated, in part, with *de novo* mutations arising in paternal germ cells," the researchers concluded.

▶ BIRTH COMPLICATIONS: Researchers have long suspected a connection between difficult deliveries and the later development of schizophrenia, but the theory is still controversial. One Swedish study published in 2001 concluded that "signs of asphyxia at birth are associated with an increased risk of schizophrenia in adults." Other studies have noted an association between early-onset schizophrenia and winter births, maternal bleeding during pregnancy, low birth weight, and complicated Caesarean deliveries.

Note that in all of the above cases, these are not yet *proven* causes, but only associations found in some clinical trials. All of the research results need to be replicated in future studies.

TARA AND TERRY-LEE MARTTINEN
A Mother and Daughter's Story

This is a tale of two generations. It's a sad story that leads to a much happier one. A story of what gets passed on, and also what changes. And it begins in 1980, in the small Northern Ontario city of Sault Ste. Marie. Terry-Lee Marttinen is sixteen years old, dating a young man named John.* Like many a teenager before her, Terry-Lee discovers she's pregnant. But at the same time, something equally unexpected is happening to John. By the time Terry-Lee announces she's having a baby, she can tell there is something wrong.

John's behaviour has become increasingly bizarre: he's smoking marijuana, dabbling in the occult. He moves out of the house. Terry-Lee is scared; she stops seeing him. But she stays in touch with his family, who is desperately trying to find help. Over the next four years, John winds up in and out of hospital, with the doctors deciding he's probably depressed. Much later – too late – they determine he's been suffering from schizophrenia all along.

One summer day in 1984, when his daughter is three, John succeeds after several attempts at suicide. He is twenty-two years old.

About a decade later, another young life is entering those delicate teen years. And Tara Marttinen is herself beginning to feel *different*. To the outside world, nothing is seriously wrong. After all, what teenager doesn't stay up late or let their grades slip slightly? In Tara, these changes are subtle enough to be virtually imperceptible. "I got a 70 in math in Grade 10," she says, "and I was an 80s student."

Then, on a day just like any other, as she sits at her desk in class, she hears, for the first time ever, a voice in her head. "It was out of the blue. I heard: 'Take off your shoes and sit under your chair.' Really loud, sort of screaming in my ear. I kind of looked around; it was maybe 9:30 in the morning when this happened." Tara is by now familiar with her father's history. She knows about the schizophrenia. "I always had the inkling in the back of my mind that it could be what my dad had. But I didn't want it to be. . . . I just figured, it's going to go away."

For the next several months she carries on with her classes, her meals with her mom, and nights out with friends as if nothing's wrong. She shares her secret with no one. But late at night, she lies awake for

---

* John is a pseudonym.

hours, unable to sleep, lost in a jumble of racing thoughts. "After a while," she says, "I knew inside. You just don't want to admit it to yourself. It's hard to."

At sixteen, partway through Grade 11, Tara finally "spills the beans" to her mother. And immediately, Terry-Lee thinks of schizophrenia. "I was always worried that maybe Tara would get it. And when she told me she was hearing voices, I knew instantly. Just instantly. My little back went up and I was instantly fearful."

We meet Terry-Lee and Tara on a sunny afternoon in May, at a bustling café in downtown Toronto. It's the start of a mini-vacation they've been planning for weeks. Together, they're visiting relatives, taking in the sights, and "shopping, shopping, shopping."

Sitting side by side, sipping tea, Tara taking one small bite of Terry-Lee's cake, it's clear that mother and daughter have an intensely symbiotic relationship. They have matching blond hair, blue-grey eyes, and friendly smiles. When one speaks, the other nods; often, they finish each other's sentences.

"We've been together a long time," Terry-Lee says proudly. "Just me and her. Being a young single mom, I think Tara and I have been really close."

Tara nods in agreement. "I actually *like* hanging out with my mom. I like sitting around watching TV with her. It's relaxing to be around someone who understands you."

Terry-Lee has bright pink lipstick, a short, spiky hairdo, and an air of happy sociability. Her daughter, she's explaining, is not big on hugs; it's one of the symptoms of her illness. So they've worked out a system for showing affection: pressing one finger to the other's shoulder. "Sometimes I just grab her anyway," Terry-Lee chuckles, demonstrating.

"She chases me around and tries to hug me," Tara says without real dismay. Tara is wafer-thin with finely carved cheekbones, alabaster skin, and a small silver hoop through her left eyebrow just above her funky black eyeglasses. Physically, she's all angles, and yet there's a softness to her, a gentle brand of confidence.

"We're very lucky," she says. "*I'm* very lucky."

Together, they want to share the story of what's made them lucky. Of how they got from there to here. *There* was Tara sitting alone in her room, writing page after page of anguished poetry:

> And my mind
> It has wings
> And is the dragon
> Setting fire
> To your dreams
> Changing everything
> Into not what it seems.

Here is Tara finishing high school with honours, Terry-Lee preparing to send her off to university. "I'm relieved," Terry-Lee says now. "When I compare Tara to her dad . . . I was so scared. And now I know it's okay. I have a safe feeling inside."

The one thing Terry-Lee knew for certain when she found out about the voices was that Tara needed help *away* from home. "I just made the assumption that the care wouldn't be any good in the Soo because of Tara's father's care. . . . There was no way I wanted that for Tara."

With a phone call to a distant uncle who worked in the field, Terry-Lee arranged an appointment at a clinic in London, seven hours away by bus. They didn't know it at the time, but what they'd stumbled into was a leading-edge treatment facility for first-episode psychosis. Dr. Ashok Malla runs the Prevention and Early Intervention Program for Psychoses, or PEPP (see page 156). Soon they were sitting in his office as he led them through a clinical assessment. Tara and Terry-Lee were each asked questions individually, then together. They both liked this doctor straight away. And straight away, he recognized the early signs of psychosis.

Before he'd even diagnosed Tara with schizophrenia, he prescribed a low dose of an atypical antipsychotic medication. "If we see symptoms, if they've been there for more than a week, we treat them," Dr. Malla says.

Tara was also given a brain scan in a magnetic resonance imaging (MRI) machine. "That was the scariest thing," she says. "But I just had this feeling: After this it's going to be better. I just knew it."

Tara was never hospitalized, never needed to be. "Thankfully," says Terry-Lee, "she never experienced the extreme changes in thinking and feelings that her father did." Instead, they returned home together to Sault Ste. Marie and went on with their lives. Tara completed Grade 11. Slowly, the voices faded away.

But other challenges remained. Schoolwork was harder than it had been, and even hanging out with friends could be exhausting. "I missed, on average, one day a week out of school. Every Thursday or Friday, just because I'd be wiped out. There was too much going on."

Tara was also tackling head-on the kind of life changes none of her friends were interested in making. Late-night drinking, dope-smoking, and partying (often staples of teenaged life in small towns, because there's not much else to do) gave way to quieter activities: jewellery-making, journal-writing, embroidery. The junk food was tossed – no more Cheez Whiz sandwiches – and replaced with a high-protein, low-sugar diet bolstered with vitamins. (Terry-Lee had done the research on the Internet.)

Twice a year, mother and daughter make the long trip to London for consultations with Dr. Malla, and Tara's medication continues to be adjusted as she copes with multiple side effects. "I have lactation," she says flatly. "That's really exciting. And allergies. You name it, I'm allergic to it now." But she doesn't have one other common side effect – weight gain – and for a young woman, that's important.

Terry-Lee, remembering what it's like to be a teenager, buys pretty containers for vitamins and medication, stocks up on herbal teas and fresh fruit, pays for art classes and Tai Chi. She's had to do some creative financing to pay for all this on her limited budget. But she feels it's important to "spend time on doing positive things to replace any losses."

If all this sounds simple, it hasn't been, as Tara wrote in a PEPP newsletter: "I have been forced to take on the huge responsibility of maintaining my own well-being. . . . I can't for even one day [diverge] from my regimen of taking my vitamins, going through my day free of over-stimulation, then taking my medication, and finally, going to bed at a decent hour. If one of these elements were missing it would have drastic effects on my performance the next day."

The payoff, however, has been huge. In five years, Tara has never had a relapse. She's become so in tune with her own mind and body that she can, in effect, stop psychosis in its tracks. "I just know when I'm not right. I know when something's wrong and when I should rest. You get to feeling dissociated, and spacey, and colours become really bright, and things like that. Over-stimulated, I guess."

"We've had to learn what those symptoms are," says Terry-Lee. "The earliest, earliest ones. Because those only require lifestyle adjustments if you catch it very early. Tara adjusts her lifestyle and then she's fine."

Doctors call these very early symptoms "prodromal," and there is much research underway into how and even if they should be treated medically. But Tara and Terry-Lee seem to have figured out how to manage them on their own.

Dr. Malla, meanwhile, is thrilled with Tara's progress. "She has a vision of her life," he says, "of what she wants to do."

What Tara wanted to do, after high school, was no different than what many kids want: to go to university. In Sault Ste. Marie, that meant leaving home – always a nerve-racking transition, but especially so for the Marttinens. "It's a creep-up-behind-you kind of disease," Terry-Lee observes. "So we're trying to be realistic. Do the homework, cover the bases, and then leap off the cliff."

That meant choosing university in London, where Dr. Malla is. It meant Tara working for a year after high school to save money, applying for student loans, and winning scholarships to help pay for tuition and books. And deciding against a room in residence – "too chaotic, too much going on," says Tara.

Today, the results of all that homework can be found on a secluded street in a remarkably homey, immaculately clean apartment at the back of an old house. This is Tara's new home, the start of her new life.

She shares it with her gerbil, Milo, who travelled with her from Sault Ste. Marie, and a rabbit called Lucy, who munches contentedly on alfalfa sprouts inside her spacious cage.

Tara has been planning this move for years, squirrelling away the contents of a home: everything from lamps to linens. Starting over has been, she says, "a lot easier than I thought it would be. I was homesick at first. But I like living on my own right now. It's very comfortable. It's my own space."

She's pacing herself carefully. Taking three classes (English Literature, Calculus, Psychology) instead of a full course-load of five. Keeping the usual first-year socializing to a minimum. "I'm a loner anyway," she says with a self-deprecating laugh.

What she misses most are the nights stretched out on the couch at home, watching TV with her mom. The bus ride costs $200, so she won't be returning until Christmas.

What she seems to like most is the quiet nest she's built for herself here. On her apartment walls, she's hung pieces of her own textile art, soon to be displayed at a PEPP exhibit. "I just show whatever I'm thinking about," she says, "whatever colour my mind is that day." She points to her latest work, which is vividly coloured with skies of pink silk, hills of purple, and a green gossamer lake replete with fish and bobbing mermaids. "It's the lake in the Soo," she explains.

In her mind's eye, Tara carries a picture of the future. As always, she has a plan: Regular visits to the PEPP clinic, where her medications will continue to be adjusted and through which she's been organizing a peer support group for young people. A summer job waitressing, perhaps at the friendly family-run restaurant she's checked out down the street. A four-year honours degree in psychology completed over five years, including summer classes and a full course-load in the final year. And after all that, a career counselling teens with mental health issues. Tara has strong feelings about stigma, and the need to break it down, and she's not shy about telling people she has a mental illness.

Even further down the road, she foresees marriage and kids, and perhaps a chance to be medication-free. "If for some reason my brain's sort-of levelled out again . . . I don't want to be on meds and having kids."

But all that is far in the future. For now, she's focused on school, on learning to "help people like me." She's making friends, but is not looking for a boyfriend – although she's clearly given it some thought. "I don't want to be with a person who doesn't respect my illness and understand the importance of it, and the place it takes in my life," she says firmly. "It's a big part of my life. I don't want it to be, but it is. It's something I have to deal with, and they would, too, as a result of being with me. So I think that's a lot of responsibility for me and for a future partner, too. And I don't think right now anybody's prepared for that."

Back at the café table, Terry-Lee shakes her head, amazed. "She's wise. She freaks me out. But I understand why she's wise. Tara's spent more time thinking about the meaning of life than most people do in a lifetime."

Tara, slightly embarrassed, allows that she has "grown up fast." But she finishes her thought in a way that reminds us she isn't *too* grown-up just yet. "It's like you're sixteen," she says, "and suddenly feel thirty, you know?"

Because the comment draws laughter from the rest of us at the table, Tara – ever considerate – adds: "Forty, eighty, whatever. More like eighty." Then, discreetly, she smiles.

Tara has now completed her first year of university. Terry-Lee promotes early intervention in every way she can.

EARLY-INTERVENTION PROGRAMS

In Canada, early-intervention programs exist in Calgary, Halifax, Hamilton, London, Montreal, Quebec City, Saskatoon, Toronto, Vancouver, and Victoria. There is no nationally organized policy or funding for these programs.

PROFILE OF PEPP

Dr. Ashok Malla is program director of the Prevention and Early Intervention Program for Psychoses (PEPP) in London, Ontario. Opened in 1997, it was one of the first early-intervention programs in Canada. A clinical and research staff of 27 people (including psychiatrists, nurses, social workers, and occupational therapists) has worked with 239 individuals to date. Most are aged sixteen to thirty.

For anyone who thinks of schizophrenia as a debilitating illness, Tara's story is heartening. And Dr. Malla says it is by no means unique. "It all depends on, are people getting the kind of help that they need?" he says. "We see this as an opportunity . . . to in fact *prevent* disability if you intervene early."

The goal is to get help for people as soon as possible after symptoms of psychosis begin. Researchers now talk about a "critical period" of five years. "I think it's now obvious that the first five years of the illness are crucial, that whatever change you can make during that period would be a lot more sustainable, and that most of the deterioration in the illness occurs in those five years," says Dr. Malla, who has conducted several research studies through PEPP. "Initially, this was a hypothesis, but I think there is enough evidence now to show that that *is* the case."

Even within those five years, the research suggests, the earlier the intervention, the better, so that young people can get back to the ordinary stuff of life.

"If you've got a seventeen-year-old, those five years are *crucial* for that person. Because it's during those five years that they're going to finish high school, go to university or get a job, have a relationship. Once you've got that stability, it's much easier to deal with whatever else is coming up."

To improve the "early" part of early intervention, PEPP runs a city-wide awareness campaign, working with local high schools and putting information packages in the orientation kits of every first-year university and college student. (London has a large student population.) They place brightly coloured posters on city buses and school bulletin boards, and produce T-shirts, brochures, and television commercials. "We have data now clearly showing we have reduced delay, in the first three years [of the campaign], by 50 per cent," Dr. Malla says.

To encourage people to visit, PEPP does assessments without a doctor's referral, and commits to seeing everyone within forty-eight hours of a phone call.

Equally important is the nature of the treatment itself. "Early intervention requires a very specialized treatment for young people. I think it's extremely important that we design treatments that they will accept and that is suitable for families."

Treatment involves low doses of the latest generation of antipsychotic medications and high doses of psychological intervention, with a case manager as well as group therapy. All this is generally done without a hospital stay. "Throughout that period, the vital thing they have going is that intense relationship with one case manager who helps them through every step. Plus, they see their psychiatrist on a regular basis to get their medication adjusted."

82 per cent of participants have completed their first year — a low drop-out rate, especially among young people.

Current funding allows for only two years of treatment, although Dr. Malla would like to extend that to five years. Because early-intervention programs are so new, there are few long-term studies to confirm what Dr. Malla and many others now believe: that appropriate treatment offered early will reap lasting health benefits.

EARLY WARNING SIGNS

Some of the early signs of psychosis Dr. Malla says are important to watch for, especially if there's a family history of mental illness, include:

▶ social withdrawal, not just from parents but from peers
▶ loss of concentration and attention abilities
▶ changes in work habits, especially loss of organizational skills
▶ a drop in school performance.

"It's the *change* that is important, in the context of having a family history," he says. "If people are noticing some substantial changes in a child's behaviour . . . *something* is going on. It may be depression. It may be something else. But there is no harm in getting it checked out. . . . It is a checkup like any other checkup."

CHAPTER 4 WHY IT HAPPENS

~m~

Oh man.

Wanna get in an argument fast? Go to a gathering of people with mental health issues and raise the topic of why people become unwell. You'll quickly discover that people have very different views on this volatile issue.

We spent an entire chapter covering this debate in our last book, but it really comes down to this: some people believe environment (abuse, poverty, dysfunction, and so on) causes mental health issues; some people believe genetics and biochemistry and neurology are to blame; and some people think there's no clear way to draw a line between the two. (You've probably noticed this in some of the stories you've read so far.)

Does a person get depressed because levels of the neuro-transmitter serotonin have dropped? Or do the levels of serotonin drop because something is deeply troubling them? Why will two people, experiencing very similar life events, react in completely different ways? Why is it that one person who tumbles down the steps fractures their ankle, while someone else takes an identical fall and walks away unharmed?

Good bones? Bad luck? Slippery steps?

The example only hints at the unbelievable complexity of *why* these things happen.

On the surface, something like posttraumatic stress disorder seems pretty clear cut: there is a cause and effect. And so it should be of little surprise that Lieutenant-General Roméo Dallaire developed vivid flashbacks after witnessing the horrors of Rwanda. And yet, like slipping on the steps, there are others who returned from that carnage and did not develop the disorder.

It gets more confusing (and volatile) when you get into the diagnosis of schizophrenia. Many sufferers grew up in good homes with good families and with no obvious "triggers." Yet there are also plenty of people who have been diagnosed with schizophrenia who endured emotional and physical abuse or trauma.

How is it possible that these very different people wound up with the same disease? Is it the same illness? (There's a growing consensus that what is currently lumped under the single label of "schizophrenia" may actually be many different disorders with different causes.)

Our approach, in this divisive field, has always been to listen to people. To let *them* explain why things happened. In doing so, we've learned that mental disorder is a highly individual experience – vastly more complex and human than the limited templates and labels we try to assign.

The stories in this chapter represent just a few of the myriad explanations people have for why it happened to them. There are, no doubt, countless more.

CARLING BASSETT-SEGUSO
The Pressures of Elite Sport

As any journalist will tell you, arranging an interview with a performer, writer, politician, athlete – anyone with even a *hint* of celebrity
– is almost always a complicated business, involving multiple phone
calls, faxes, and negotiations with assistants, agents, or secretaries.

Not so with Carling Bassett-Seguso.

"Sure," she says brightly when we call. Through her cellphone, we
hear tennis balls thudding against racquets; she's just stepped off the
practice courts. "How about right now?"

Fiddling with tape recorder, scrambling to find notes, we reschedule
for early the next morning. From her home in the affluent beach
and tennis community of Boca Raton, Florida, in a conversation punctuated by probing questions from her three young children – "Mom,
what does *Scandinavian* mean?" – she happily answers several dozen
questions about anorexia, bulimia, and life as a young tennis star.

"I'm very open about myself. A lot of people say, 'You really
shouldn't be,' but it doesn't bother me. If I can help one person, then
it gives me such gratification. Because it's horrifying. To be in that
place in your life – nobody wants to be there."

Bassett-Seguso is proof personified that mental disorder knows no
boundaries of wealth, talent, or personality. Because from birth, she's
had all of these things in spades. As a teenager, her sunny disposition,
combined with California-girl good looks and a penchant for pounding unreturnable tennis balls across a net, made her the media darling
of her sport. Known to drive grown men gaga, "Darling Carling" was
the 1980s precursor to Anna Kournikova but without the 'tude.
"Carling Bassett's life might have been conjured up by a genie who
decided to give her all the wishes she wanted," one star-struck (male)
reporter wrote in a 1986 article, listing her favourite things as "boys,
shopping and fast cars."

If reminder ever need be served that humans are far more complex
than the images we project, here's what was happening when that
story was written: eighteen-year-old Carling was putting her fingers

down her throat and throwing up on a daily basis. She was caught in a binge-and-purge cycle that ultimately ended her career as a professional tennis player.

It was another, older tennis player who showed Carling how to induce vomiting. She was fifteen then, and had just broken into the big leagues on the women's circuit, reaching her first tournament final, where she took top seed Chris Evert to three sets. Off the courts, she had the same preoccupations as most other teenage girls.

"At that time I had my first boyfriend, and I just wanted to be thinner. Maybe because so much was put upon me. I remember eating Oreos and just feeling so guilty. And trying to put my finger down my throat, but nothing really came up. And then it's like any kind of disease – it progresses slowly."

Many a teenage tennis sensation has succumbed, either physically or emotionally, to the demands of instant celebrity – think Jennifer Capriati (in her early tennis career) or Andrea Jaeger. But Carling Bassett seemed better-equipped than most to handle the pressure. Her father, John Bassett Jr., had himself been a professional tennis player; he'd also owned several professional sports teams. Both her parents were wealthy beyond belief – her mother's ancestors founded the Carling brewery while her father came from a long line of media magnates. The whole family was used to the spotlight. "I always had a lot of publicity even before I exploded onto the women's tour," Bassett-Seguso says. "My dad was a very prominent businessman and sports figure, and liked the publicity. We grew up from a very young age being exposed to it. So I always felt comfortable with it."

She was also, by the time of her first tournament final, accustomed to winning, and to a highly competitive environment. From the age of eleven, she'd lived and trained at the world-renowned Bollettieri Tennis Academy, where the likes of Andre Agassi and Monica Seles later started out. "I wasn't at all near the level [the other kids] played at. So it was good, because with my competitive nature, I wanted to achieve that type of success. I worked very very hard and I did have a lot of natural ability. I could learn quickly."

Did she ever. At thirteen, she was the top women's player in Canada. At fourteen, she hoisted the coveted Orange Bowl trophy for juniors, which de facto made her the top female player in the world under eighteen. Soon after, she turned pro full-time. Today, under WTA (Women's Tennis Association) rules, that wouldn't be allowed. But in 1983, young talents routinely went full-swing onto the women's tour long before they could drive or drink. Bassett-Seguso still thinks it was the right choice for her. "I had done everything [as a junior]. There wasn't really anywhere else for me to go."

Very quickly, she earned her place. That first year on the tour, the WTA named her Most Impressive Newcomer. The next year, she reached her first Grand Slam semi-final, at the U.S. Open. And just as quickly, the media came calling. As so often happens, athletic success commingled with beauty and charisma to create a dynamic driven not by sport, but by money and marketing. Soon, young Carling had acquired a management team and a contract with the prestigious Ford Models agency. She did fashion shoots and commercials for C-Plus, Canada Dry, McDonald's. She had her own line of sportswear and starred in a movie, *Spring Fever*. She even guest-starred as herself on a network soap opera.

"That's where I think things started to get a little messy," she recalls today. "Oh my God! It was like a whirlwind . . . you want to please and impress. . . . And I'm around all those models. And when you have that obsessive-compulsive, very driven personality, you want to be great in every area. And then I think you just kind of lose control."

Somehow, amidst all the hype and despite her ongoing bulimia, her game kept improving. In 1985, at seventeen, she reached a career-high ranking of eighth in the world. No Canadian has ever ranked higher. Achieving that level of play meant intensive training, which made her physically hungry. It also meant extensive travel, with a new tournament, another faceless hotel room, every week. Lonely at the end of a long day, Carling turned to food – "chocolate, bread . . . I didn't know a whole lot about nutrition" – and then, inevitably, to purging.

"That's what I could really control. So much of everything that went on around me was *out* of my control. People made decisions for me. I was pulled in so many different directions. And there was so much pressure to always do well."

The sad irony of eating disorders is that the search for control results in its opposite. And while she continued touring, picking up her racquet and smiling for the cameras, teenage Carling's illness became progressively worse. "It becomes more frequent. I remember one time purging all day long to the point where it's *water* [coming up]. You're bloated all the time. I remember one time waking up at two in the morning and – how crazy is this? – I ordered a large pizza. Just woke up and decided I was going to." Eating disorders, she now believes, are like an addiction, a bad habit like smoking or drinking that, once begun, can take on a life of its own. "It just became a terrible habit, and then this habit was just my everyday way of life, and I couldn't stop. It became like a craving or an obsession or a compulsion."

Much later, in psychotherapy sessions, she would plumb the depths of her childhood and conclude that no hidden trauma lay there. She'd never lacked for self-esteem. But the travelling life kept her away from close friends and family who might have intervened. And to the rest of the world, Carling Bassett looked like a vision of health. Years of binging and purging had slowed her metabolism so much she stopped losing weight. "The most deceiving thing about a long period of bulimia is that I maintained a weight of 130 pounds, so people thought I was better. But in actual reality, that was probably when I was throwing up the most."

When Carling was eighteen and at the height of her game, her father was diagnosed with cancerous brain tumours. It was John Bassett Jr. who'd first put a tennis racquet into Carling's hands, hoping his seven-year-old would learn to love the game as passionately as he did. He'd taught her himself at first, with lessons three times a week, which young Carling had dreaded. "Tennis was *so* important to him. I never even watched tennis then. I mean, I didn't *love* tennis." Recognizing her talent, he'd encouraged his reluctant daughter – who would've preferred a pony – to give Bollettieri's a try. And there, in Florida, surrounded by players her own age, she'd started to love the game.

John Bassett Jr. died in May 1986 at the age of forty-seven. Less than two weeks later, Carling showed up at the French Open. "I have been so depressed," she told the *Los Angeles Times*, "that I just kept on playing tennis." She reached the quarter-finals that year – an emotional tribute to her father – but it would be her last real run at a Grand Slam title. At eighteen, with her eating disorder still virulent, she'd peaked as a tennis player.

At nineteen, she married Wimbledon doubles champ Robert Seguso, and at twenty she had their first child, Holden John. While pregnant, she desperately tried to control her bulimia. "I'd stopped for like two and a half, three months. And then it came back, but not as badly. And then after I had Holden, my weight dropped dramatically, because I was really fighting it. That's when I kind of slipped into the anorexia."

Suddenly removed from the rigorous travel-and-training routine, she lost her appetite entirely. In her mind, eating was by now inseparable from throwing up; anxious to give up one, she virtually abandoned the other. "I would eat the same thing every day. I would eat a little melon in the morning. Lunch would be *lettuce*." She also exercised obsessively, jogging with Holden in his stroller, preparing for a tennis comeback. And all the while, she was hiding her illness from everyone.

"Carling says she's healthy, faster than ever, although not as strong," the *Washington Post* reported at a tournament in 1989, less than a year after Holden's birth. "She's so trim, a bit thin actually, almost bony." Carling told the reporter she'd been doing sit-ups, "hundreds a day, to get rid of that stomach flab." And it had obviously, painfully, worked.

That year, at the U.S. Open – the site of her teen Grand Slam breakthrough – her weight hovered around 100 pounds. She lost in the first round. And the rumours were everywhere. The *Toronto Star* noted that Carling was "virtually a shell of her former self, physically," with a "very thin and drawn" face. Bassett-Seguso blamed the stress of new motherhood and moving house, saying her metabolism had "shot up." Her husband told the media that Carling had "always been a light eater."

"You're not going to believe this," she says now, "but my husband never even knew." In more than two years together, she had managed to keep her disordered eating from her husband. "All people with addictions, we have so many great masks. We're the best at hiding things."

The beginning of the end came in 1990, on a trip to another tennis tournament with her husband and eighteen-month-old baby. "I had a terrible, terrible anxiety attack. I said to Rob that I thought I was having a heart attack. It wasn't a heart attack. But he had to rush me to the hospital. And then I just flooded it all out, right then and there. I thought I was going to die."

It was the fear of death that got her eating again – that and "sheer will." Often, she'd wake in the night to another terrifying anxiety attack. "I was so scared of eating," she says. "I was so in fear of expelling."

Her second pregnancy – she weighed ninety-eight pounds when it began – gave her the final impetus. She started reading about eating disorders, talking to her friends, and seeing a therapist. Unlike many people with eating disorders, she was never hospitalized, and was able to recover with little professional help. "Slowly but surely, I just got better."

For the former sports star, getting better meant giving up her profession, the game she had learned to love. Disorder and tennis were, for her, inextricably intertwined: Anorexia and bulimia had prevented her from reaching the top, and competing at the top had prevented her from becoming well. "It was a huge trigger for me," she says. She now believes she could never have recovered while on the tour.

Today, Bassett-Seguso maintains an interest in her sport, playing charity events, guest-hosting on TSN, and practising with her two sons, who've become competitive tennis players themselves. (Her daughter prefers ballet.) But the once headline-making "Darling" of tennis has long since chosen a quieter life for herself. It has, she believes, been the key to her well-being. "I lead a very, very simple life. I have the most incredible husband in the world, who is so supportive of everything, and he's very non-judgmental. He's just got such a good balance. He never pushed me. I think that I've always felt like I've been pushed."

Today, she's a healthy, if still trim, 115 pounds. "I'm a fit slim," she says. "I like being that – I won't deny that. I would have trouble being heavy. I don't think that'll ever leave me. But I'm very healthy." And to remain healthy, she knows, she must be vigilant. "You always have to be on your toes and aware that it's right behind you, saying, 'Come on, let's go.'"

The teenager whose life had once spun so fast that she believed she'd never live to thirty has now beaten her own odds. Life today does not spin but rather sprints along at a fast yet manageable pace. At thirty-four, Carling Bassett-Seguso hasn't exactly slowed down. One suspects she never will. "I'm always high," she complains. "That's my problem."

But it is also her blessing, one that helps keep eating disorders at bay. "I have so much in my life now," she says quickly. "I look at my children, and they're the most important things in my life. And my husband. And I'm so busy, so active. I don't think I'd have the time."

The interview concluded, she has just five minutes to get her son to the dentist on time. When she hangs up the phone, she'll be off and out the door. She will, she says, be "going, going, going" all day long.

OTHER ATHLETES WHO'VE GONE PUBLIC

Carling Bassett-Seguso says that professional tennis now requires so much strength and power that it's unlikely many tour players have eating disorders. But these disorders continue to be a problem in other sports, such as gymnastics. Over the years, several elite athletes have gone public, including one of Bassett-Seguso's contemporaries.

▶ Tennis player Zina Garrison suffered from bulimia for many years while on the tour in the 1980s. A Wimbledon finalist and top-five player, she would later tell the *San Francisco Chronicle* that she had once "lost to someone ranked 350th in the world and I lost because I didn't have any energy."

▶ Swimmer Tiffany Cohen, who won two Olympic gold medals in 1984, later became severely ill with bulimia, ending her competitive career. "Instead of training for the '88 Olympics," she told *Sports Illustrated for Women* in 2001, "I thought of myself as lucky to be alive to watch."

▶ In the late 1970s and early 1980s, champion diver Megan Neyer suffered from eating disorders. She later said many other divers did too. "We didn't eat for three days, then we'd eat, then purge," she told the *Washington Post* in 1988. "It happened because of a win-at-all-costs attitude."

▶ Kathy Johnson, a gymnast and bronze medallist at the 1984 Olympics, was bulimic for ten years while she competed. "The problem is every athlete is somewhat compulsive," she told the San Francisco *Examiner* in 1992. "You have to be to do all the work we do."

▶ Christy Henrich, a U.S. gymnast, was 4'10" and weighed just sixty-one pounds when she died of organ failure caused by anorexia. She was twenty-two. Her mother has said that Christy's disorder started after a gymnastics judge told her she was too heavy to make the Olympic team.

ATHLETES AND EATING DISORDERS

▶ A report by the Canadian Academy of Sport Medicine warns that female athletes are at greatest risk in aesthetic sports that involve subjective judging (gymnastics, figure skating, diving, synchronized swimming) or that encourage low body weight for athletic reasons or appearance. Other studies have noted that sports that involve wearing tight-fitting outfits also see higher rates of eating disorders.

▶ A 1999 study of more than 1,400 U.S. college athletes found that 9 per cent of the females had "clinically significant problems with bulimia" and just under 3 per cent with anorexia. About 5.5 per cent reported purging with laxatives or diuretics, or vomiting at least once a week (as did 2 per cent of the males). The highest rates were among female gymnasts.

▶ A survey of elite distance runners in Britain found that 16 per cent of the women had an eating disorder at the time of the study. This group had a lower body-mass index, lower self-esteem, and poorer mental health than the runners without an eating disorder.

▶ A University of Georgia study of twenty-five female gymnasts found that 61 per cent had not had a menstrual cycle in three or more months.

▶ Another study tracking the diets of forty junior-level competitive figure skaters found that "inadequate energy intakes and delayed menarche (in women) were widespread."

ALLAN STRONG
"Is It in the Genes?"

My first experience with mental illness came when I was eleven years old. I had always suspected there was something wrong with my mother, but my suspicions were confirmed when she kept myself, my brother, and my two sisters home from school because there was a holy war being fought in the streets outside of our home. My mother believed that she was God's messenger here on Earth and that she was directing the forces of good in the struggle against the forces of evil. I can remember trying to reassure my younger siblings that everything would be all right as soon as Dad got home. But I was frightened and could not understand what was happening.

My father was a salesman and was away for a few days. We ended up missing a week of school. During that time, we all had to sleep in sleeping bags huddled around the fireplace. (Mom believed that the rest of the house wasn't safe from the forces of evil.) Unfortunately, what was fuelling the fire in the fireplace were books and family photos, which Mom thought were satanic. When Dad got home, she was hospitalized.

I spent my adolescence walking on eggshells. When my mother was well, she was very competent. An active community volunteer all her life, she did telephone outreach for a number of community groups, volunteered with the local AIDS committee, and was the local representative for a support group for parents of lesbian and gay youth. She always had a lot of friends. But when she was sick she was completely unpredictable. Like a lot of people in similar circumstances, Mom would drink and become verbally abusive.

It would have been nice if the "system" had offered some acknowledgement of our family's struggles. I think my parents had a few joint sessions with her psychiatrist, but nothing was made available to us children. And we often had to endure her illness alone while Dad was on the road.

I didn't feel there was anyone outside the home I could talk to, and most of my friends did not understand. A girlfriend in high school actually asked me if it was something she could catch. In hindsight, this statement might have been prophetic, as I did catch it: I was diagnosed with bipolar disorder in my mid-thirties.

For most of my adult life, I was called upon to clean up the mess caused by Mom's frequent episodes. By the time I left home to work in Toronto, she was averaging one hospitalization a year. She finally did get settled into a medication routine that seemed to work for her; it was only then that our relationship began to resemble a normal mother-son relationship.

My mother died when I was thirty-five. I had been seeing her quite regularly. I was married, and Mom was quite impressed by my wife and held her in very high esteem. She also really enjoyed seeing our son, Jacob, and relished the time she spent with him. Her death caught me off-guard, and the next year was a whirlwind of trying to settle her estate, sell her house, and maintain peace between the four of us kids. Once the estate was finally settled, I slowly went to pieces.

At first I had difficulty getting to sleep. Then I wouldn't have the energy to get out of bed. I felt like I was on a roller coaster. I was bad-tempered and argumentative; in short, I was very difficult to be around. Thus my second encounter with the mental health system began not as a family member but as a consumer.

I had always wondered if one of us kids would get ill, but I didn't expect it to be me. For some bizarre reason I thought I was immune because I worked in social services. (I suppose I went into the field because I was used to being a helper; as a professional, I could play out the caregiver role I had been in since I was young.) I had, by this point, worked in the mental health field for almost ten years, so I knew what a mood disorder was. I had been the president of the Depressive and Manic-Depressive Association of Ontario, and had given numerous presentations about mental illness, but always from a family member's perspective. I even knew there was some research to suggest that these illnesses might run in families. But I never once thought that I would get ill.

In hindsight, though, I had been dealing with depression for most of my life. I just always managed to cope. I also now realize that I self-medicated with alcohol. When I got to feeling blue, I would drown my sorrows in a bottle or two. In my naïveté I didn't make the connection, or chose not to.

When Mom died, the usual defences didn't work any more; I fell to pieces over a four-month span, slowly deteriorating to the point where I was unable to function at all. I stayed up all night imagining people were hiding in the house waiting to get me. During the day, I wandered from room to room looking for intruders. I stopped going to work. Later, my wife, Sue, told me she was afraid that she would come home from work and find me dead. That was her worst fear, and she didn't know what to do about it.

I made a half-hearted attempt at suicide, which brought me to a hospital and introduced me to the mental health world from a different perspective. Some things hadn't changed; I was taken to the hospital by ambulance with Sue following by car. From the start, all the attention was brought to bear on me, the patient, while my wife, the caregiver, received none. Actually, there was one support group for families at the hospital, but it was held from three to four in the afternoon – not a good time for a working mother.

My diagnosis helped explain some of the things I had long been feeling. However, as the label sank in, my worst fear was that I would end up like my mother. I had seen what years of strong medication had done to her. And I had seen what accepting a label of "mentally ill person" had done to her expectations of herself.

I did not want to live my life that way. But part of me was afraid that I would have to settle for less than I was used to expecting of myself and for myself.

In total, I have been hospitalized three times. My son was just past a year old when I was first hospitalized. When I was recovering at home from my second hospitalization, he asked me why I was so scared all the time. Jacob also began to tell us about having dreams of men in white coats coming to take his daddy away. We did the best we could to reassure him, but as a family we did not know where to turn for the answers to his concerns. The mental health system has done a lousy job of responding to our needs for nurture, support, and relief – it wasn't there for me as a child, and it has certainly not been there for my family.

I have worked in mental health for close to twenty years, I have seen first-hand the incredible toll that mental health issues can take on a family, and I have personally struggled with my own demons. What have I learned from all this?

I now have to wonder if my becoming ill was a result of lousy genes, learned behaviour, environmental stress, or a combination of all three. On the genetics side of the equation, my mother was bipolar, and my mother's father was kept out of the armed forces during the Second World War due to a diagnosis of "dementia praecox," which was an early term for what is now called schizophrenia. I don't know if my mother's father *had* schizophrenia, but he was certainly very paranoid. I'm also told that my father's father suffered from episodes of deep depression.

Or perhaps I responded to life in a certain way because of what I saw and learned from my mother. Then again, I became ill the year after my mother died, so maybe environmental factors played a part? I've come to believe that we all have genetic predispositions, but these are triggered by cues from the environment. I feel that I may have a predisposition to depression, but that being raised as I was con- tributed to me becoming bipolar. If things were different in my house, I might not have developed anything.

I am blessed to have a supportive and caring spouse and family, and part of that family has been an extremely supportive church that has stood by me.

I have promised myself that I am never going to refer to myself as "bipolar." My mother lived that label, defining herself by her diagnosis. Often, she would say, "What do you expect from a manic-depressive?" I don't want that label, and I am not going to allow myself to be limited by any diagnosis someone else has given me.

I have learned that no matter what happens to me, I will always be honest and truthful with both my children about what is happening.

(I also have a younger daughter, born after my hospitalizations.) My wife and I want them to understand what I go through and not to be afraid. They know that Daddy needs to take pills to be well, and when he is not well he sleeps a lot. I know that my illness affects my children, because they notice when I am not doing well (which usually means that I am in bed for the whole weekend or I yell at them). We try to talk about it, and we try to carry on as well as we can.

I think about my own children and I wonder how their will lives be. Will they be touched with depression or bipolar disorder or schizophrenia? Will the genetic links that seem to run through our family touch their lives as they have touched mine? While writing this, I have been thinking about what I would do if one of my children did develop a mental illness. I have been asked, in the past, if I regret having children, since my family history suggests a strong genetic predisposition to a mood disorder. My answer is that I do not for one minute regret having our children. They have been a gift from the Almighty and they have done more to make my life worth living than anything else possibly could.

As a society we have to learn to accept that, no matter what label we give them, people still have abilities and skills. My children, if they do develop a mental illness, will still be the beautiful people that God intended them to be. I like to believe that the work I do will help to make a difference for them. If I can leave any type of legacy to them it would be the ability to challenge the myths and labels that society gives us and to be who they want to be no matter what.

If my children do happen to struggle with a mental disorder, will the world be a more tolerant and understanding place?

I hope and pray that it will be.

Allan Strong works for the Wellness Network, a consumer-survivor organization in Southwestern Ontario.

WISE WORDS

The Canadian Mental Health Association conducted a survey of family members affected by depression and bipolar disorder, including adult children who had a parent with a mood disorder. The resulting booklet, called *Hear Me Now*, offers advice that applies to any mental disorder, including this: "Children will notice that something is amiss in their family and will try to make sense of it. The trouble is, the explanations kids come up with on their own may be incorrect. . . . So, while it may not be easy, it is important to keep children in the loop when a parent suffers from a mood disorder. . . . The basic message is this: Daddy [or Mommy] isn't feeling well. He feels very sad; it's because of an illness and it's not anybody's fault. It is a sad time for all of us, but I'm here to talk to you about it when you need to."

DONNA MORRISSEY
A Medical Scare

Donna Morrissey has her life's work down to a manageable routine now. In the morning, she writes. Then she heads to the gym, stops for lunch, and gets back to the computer for a second stretch of writing that often reaches into the early evening.

We catch up with her right after the gym section of the day, and Morrissey is brimming with all kinds of positive energy. Dressed in cargo pants, a striped red T-shirt, and a floppy brimmed hat, sunglasses slung round her neck on a black rope, she looks tireless and young – unnaturally young for her forty-five years. She's chosen a busy little café near her home in downtown Halifax, and, it seems, she knows both menu and staff exceptionally well; she cheers and high-fives the young woman who ducks into the kitchen to find one last remaining date cookie for her.

"I *love* these cookies," Morrissey says happily, her eyes a brilliant green.

It was a friend who suggested Morrissey try writing fiction, saying, "If you can write like you talk . . ." One can easily see why the comment was made. The woman tells a tale with flourish, arms flying through the air, bum shifting in her seat. Words come out rapid-fire and full of every conceivable emotion. "The biggest shock on leaving my outport was discovering the queer way that everybody spoke!" she says with her now muted Newfoundland brogue. "The way they all looked at me when I didn't speak *clearly*."

Morrissey's first novel, *Kit's Law*, is set in a tiny Newfoundland outport most easily accessible by boat, not unlike the place where she grew up. And from the sounds of it, The Beaches was an idyllic place to be a kid. "Everybody's door was open. Everybody had a hand in smacking you across the arse if we went too far, or near the water. . . . There was the ocean in front of you, and the woods in the back, and they were your parameters. And in between was your mother and your grandmothers and your aunts and your uncles."

As most young people do, Morrissey left The Beaches. At sixteen, having flunked out of high school, she set off travelling that vast expanse of country to the west. "I was like, 'Jesus, I want to see a hippie! And I want to smoke pot, and I want to do all of that stuff and travel the world.' I didn't do the world so much, but I certainly traipsed through this country a few times."

For ten years, Morrissey moved from province to province, working as a waitress, a bartender, a cook on an oilrig. She got married and had two children (a son, now twenty-six, and a daughter, now nineteen). And when she tired of life "abroad," she brought her family back to Newfoundland and worked splitting cod at a fish processing plant. It was there, in St. John's, when Donna Morrissey was thirty-two, that crisis struck.

It started with some bad fish and the plant advising all its workers, as a precaution, to get a tetanus shot. Morrissey happened to be going home for a holiday that week, so decided to have the shot there. "The doctor lived right next to my mom, so I just thought I'd hop over and get that done. And while I was in there saying I needed a tetanus shot, he looked at my hand and he saw some little cuts. And he said, 'Are you experiencing any kind of stiffness of your neck or throat?' And I'd just spent fifteen hours on a bus getting home, and I said, 'Well, yes, I am, as a matter of fact.'"

After checking her pulse and examining her throat, the conversation went something like this:

Doctor:	You have tetanus.
Morrissey:	Okay. So what do we do now?
Doctor:	Nothing. It's lethal. You have at most six months to live.

Some fifteen years later, Morrissey has instant recall of that moment. She can still see herself there, in abject terror, sitting in a chair in that small, sterile clinic. "That was the moment for me. The moment that can never ever be undone. . . . He said those words – 'it's lethal' – and everything left me. All reason left me. All I felt was this incredible sensation of sinking, losing, swimming, my stomach overwhelming me with its feelings of total fear."

It's the moment she blames – and it still makes her mad – for the anxiety, panic, and phobias that invaded her life for many years to come. It's the moment that triggered unwanted memories.

Years earlier, when Donna Morrissey was twenty-three, she had held her father's best friend as he died of a heart attack. A few months later, her own best friend died in an accident. And in between these two terrifying events, something far worse. Her younger brother died in a work-related accident while he and Donna were living and working in Alberta. "When you're twenty-three years old and you're so far away from home, and you've dealt with this kind of tragedy, and you've got to take this home to your mom and dad, things happen that you don't know how to process, really. So when this doctor told me that it was my turn to die, he triggered trauma that was so set within me that I really hadn't learned to express it."

Morrissey was told she could die at any moment. The doctor, someone Donna had not previously met, sent her home with pills to take in case of an attack that very night. And he instructed her to get to the nearest hospital the next morning. One can imagine the kind of night that must have been.

At the hospital, after a thorough work-up, she was told there'd been some kind of mistake; she was, in fact, perfectly healthy. The doctors suggested she go home and throw herself a party. Which she did. "I had a great big party, a three-day party. . . . And when I went back to St. John's, after the holiday was over, I resumed normal living." Then she adds firmly: "There *is* such a thing as normal – I now know that, because I've never been normal since. So I know what was normal before that."

Morrissey went back to work at the plant. She took care of her kids, spent time with friends. Then in the early hours one morning, just after some of her closest friends had said goodnight, everything crumbled. "I was just doing that last-minute cleanup before you go to bed so you don't have to deal with the empties in the morning . . . and I was walking up the stairs to go to bed. Just skipping up the stairs, and suddenly it was like something hit me, something black and awful, like I'd hit a wall. It was that sudden, and it was that physical. It brought me to my knees. . . . I crawled upstairs, got into bed, and finally I went to sleep. And when I woke up – *wham*, there it was again. I walked around like that for eight months."

During those eight months of "black, dark, awful" fear and anxiety, Morrissey told no one what she was feeling. She said she was fine, if ever anyone cared to ask. Went to work each day, came home again each night, all on a kind of auto-pilot. "And all I kept thinking about was, 'Jesus, I'm mad, this is madness!' and I knew it totally had to do with that doctor."

Finally, one morning as she was driving to work, she found herself so exhausted she could no longer go through the motions. "All of my energy was being taken trying to cope with feelings of fear inside of me, and fear for no reason. I just felt choked in fear, and I couldn't break away from it." In desperation, Morrissey drove, in full fish-worker's gear, to a doctor's office in St. John's.

"I'll never forget the moment. I was wearing a white coat, rubber boots, and I had a hairnet on, and a splitting-knife tucked into my rubber boot. And I just pulled my car over, got out of the car, walked into his office." She told the doctor she thought she was going crazy. She started to cry. Then the doctor leaned forward in his chair and did something entirely unexpected. He handed her a lollipop. "A candy sucker! And he pulled one out for himself, and he said, 'Oh, do you really think so?' And I remember saying, 'Just when I thought I'd had every kind of day.'" (Years later, she would recreate elements of the scene in *Kit's Law*.)

Then another odd thing happened. "I saw a picture of an old woman on his desk. And I said, 'She looks like my great-aunt Emma,' and he said, 'Well, her name is Emma.' And it turned out we were cousins, me and the doctor. I had no idea." Not what you expect when for the first time in your life you admit to fear of losing your mind. But not entirely ineffective either. Morrissey got herself to work that day.

Meanwhile, the doctor/cousin referred her to a psychiatrist, then a psychologist, both of whom recommended psychotherapy. It didn't help her much. "The psychiatrist was bloody well learned, wasn't she, and the psychologist was bloody well learned," Morrissey says, her face switching from humorous-scene-telling mode to a flush of real anger. "They looked at me and said, 'We don't think you've resolved your grief around your brother.' I [thought] 'Don't give me that shit – maybe I haven't, but where's my pill and where's my cure? I've seen a lot of people in grief but I don't see them walking around like me.' I sound really cynical and I am, because they didn't help me."

What did help was a book recommended by her psychiatrist on Morrissey's very last visit. "She had little else to say to me that day, and her eyes just happened to fall on this book that some other poor idiot left behind the last time they sat in the chair I was now sitting in." The book was called *Hope and Help for Your Nerves*, and reading it was a profound experience. In it, she discovered such terms as "generalized anxiety" and "posttraumatic stress disorder," both of which she concluded applied to her.

Intrigued, she started taking psychology courses, and five years later she had earned a social work degree from Memorial University. (She got divorced during this time, too.)

"I started piecing together what happened to me back there and understanding. Then I was able to at least work with it." Where she had once stayed silent, she now started telling anyone and everyone about what ailed her, soliciting opinions and advice. "I found my information through friends, through talking my heart out . . . and through reading, through my own research," she says. In this regard, she considers herself fortunate.

"What causes me suffering," she says, picking up speed and fury like a preacher at the pulpit, "is knowing that in those outports where I come from – and in these tiny little towns all over the country – there are so many people who suffer in silence; they still don't have what I have found in terms of support and knowledge. They're cut off from that."

Read as she could, talk as she might, Morrissey's own troubles were far from over. Anxiety plagued her for years, worse at some times than others, but never really disappearing. "No matter how hard I worked with it, it wouldn't end. It was always there. It was like a fucking bird flying over my head, with its shadow. Even though you might be anxiety-free for today or this week or this month, even, you never felt that it wasn't going to catch up with you. So you become afraid of lots of things. You don't want to travel. You don't want to go far from home. I never did become agoraphobic, but I certainly see how that can happen."

Morrissey, who had travelled the country solo as a teenager, hitch-hiking and camping and fearing nothing, now found herself terrified by a twenty-minute bus ride across town. Sitting close by the exit, she'd try to protect herself against . . . "What? I don't know. The past, the fear you'd freak out in front of [people], whatever."

An anxiety disorder, she came to understand, is nothing like your occasional, run-of-the-mill bout of nervousness. "Patterns of thought become entrenched; patterns of being, of thinking. It changed everything about me: how I thought, how I saw things, what I did, everything." Getting others to understand these concepts was another matter. When she told a boyfriend she was struggling with anxiety, he suggested a walk. "It's like, 'Sweetheart, I went for 5,000 walks! I've walked 5 million miles! This isn't about taking a walk!' Unless they've been there, I don't think they really understand."

Morrissey describes anxiety as a physical presence, a bodily experience she equates to a car engine grinding because it lacks oil. When she read up on serotonin depletion and its possible effects on the brain and emotions, the physicality made sense to her. "I could just feel my brain grind with no fucking grease in it! And it was like, Would somebody loosen it, free it, oil it? But I couldn't find anybody with intelligence enough to put it together for me."

If the ineffectual doctors prolonged her agony, and the confluence of traumatic events preceded and contributed to it, Morrissey still lays the bulk of blame at the feet of that outport doctor who'd told her she would die. "*He* made me sick. I'm sure if he had said that to my mother, it wouldn't have happened. So [there is] a predisposition, maybe, [but] he was the trigger."

University helped, because it gave her a routine and an incentive to keep getting up every day. But recovery was "clawing, day by day, week by week, month by month."

Morrissey started writing after finishing her degree, taking pen and paper to a neighbourhood café each morning. Not long after, she moved to Halifax, where she wrote seven hours a day: short stories, screenplays. She was in her late thirties and only just discovering where her talents, and her passions, lay. And very quickly, she was winning awards and critical acclaim.

When her mother – "my heroine" – was diagnosed with terminal cancer, Donna Morrissey moved back to The Beaches to care for her. There, by her mother's bedside, and with her input and advice, she wrote the manuscript for *Kit's Law*, telling the story of a teenage girl growing up in a troubled home in an outport called Haire's Hollow. When the manuscript was finished, they mailed it off and anxiously waited – together, because it was a labour of their shared love – for an acceptance letter. In the months ahead, while her mother's health deteriorated, there would be no such letter. And soon her mother was at death's door. Then another striking confluence of events, which Morrissey later described in print: "Sunday, at 2 p.m., she departed.

Monday, at 9 a.m., Penguin Canada called. My mother had plied the hand of God, and I was now a writer."

The novel became a national bestseller, winning a Canadian Booksellers Association award and being picked up by publishers in Europe, Japan, and the United States. Its success – *her* success – has in turn forced Donna Morrissey to take the final plunge in overcoming her anxiety. "Suddenly, I had to go on this cross-Canada tour, and I had to do public readings. I am phobic of flying. I have a phobia of public speaking. I had like twelve ongoing phobias, and I had to now do this solo act. And I thought, 'There's not a chance in hell.' But at the same time, I said, 'There's not a chance in hell that I'm missing it, either. No way. It's too exciting.'"

A close friend encouraged Morrissey to try an anti-anxiety drug called Celexa, which had worked wonders for her. Morrissey, who had "started getting tired of the fight," decided to give the little white pill a try.

"Gee, it was hard. I remember standing there with that little pill in my hand for two, three, maybe four or five days, trying to get the courage to swallow it. Finally, I had to. I was going across the country, alone, flying, reading to 400 people in Vancouver. So I just had to."

Several nights into her tour, she found herself coming to a realization: *nothing was going to go wrong*. She's stayed on the drug ever since, although now at a reduced dose. "I'll never go off it," she says.

Since that tour, Morrissey has published a second novel, *Downhill Chance*, also set in Newfoundland. She's travelled to England, navigating the London Underground alone, appearing on live television and radio – something that can raise the blood pressure of even the calmest soul – without a hitch. The medication "works beautifully. I do my presentations and my talks, and I go anywhere I want." When she travels now, she carries a pill in her pocket, a few in her purse, and more in her suitcase. "It's like, don't let me be separated!"

Soon she'll be off to New York, the first of several stops promoting *Kit's Law* in the United States. And this time, there's no anxious waiting for a publisher for her new book: she already has three – one for Canada, another for the United States, and a third for Britain.

"I want to cross my fingers and say, 'Jesus! Don't go singing too loud, because the song might end tomorrow,'" she says, laughing. "When you go through these feelings of fear and anxiety, you start understanding we're so vulnerable – you don't take anything for granted."

And she doesn't.

ANXIETY DISORDERS

▶ Worldwide, anxiety disorders affect an estimated 400 million people at any given time (World Health Organization).

▶ Anxiety disorders are the most prevalent mental disorders among adults (U.S. Surgeon General's report on mental health).

▶ The best estimate reached by the U.S. Surgeon General's report on mental health in the United States is that 16.4 per cent of the population has an anxiety disorder (including posttraumatic stress disorder, panic disorder, and obsessive-compulsive disorder) in any given year.

▶ Anxiety disorders affect twice as many women as men (U.S. Surgeon General's report).

▶ In 2000, Canadians made 4,563,000 visits to doctors' offices for anxiety disorders – the fifth most common reason after hypertension, depression, diabetes, and acute upper respiratory infection (IMS Health).

▶ "Anxiety disorders are among the most prevalent mental health problems experienced by Canadians. Although effective treatment approaches exist for these disorders, research suggests that mental health and health care professionals often lack appropriate knowledge about effective treatments, and may use treatments with little empirical support" (Health Canada, 1996).

"SEPTEMBER 11" SYNDROME

Most of us watched the scene in New York with horror on September 11 – either on live broadcasts or on endless repeats. Two jets, two towers, thousands of lives. Although they weren't the only commercial airliners to crash that day, they were the ones captured on tape.

In the immediate aftermath, mental health professionals were predicting a tremendous potential for posttraumatic stress disorder (PTSD), with people closest to the attacks facing increased risk.

In late March of 2002, a study published in the *New England Journal of Medicine* estimated that more than 150,000 residents of Manhattan suffered PTSD or depression following the attack.

"Given the scope of this disaster, the high prevalence of mental health problems we documented among residents of Manhattan is not surprising," said Dr. Sandro Galea, a scientist at the New York Academy of Medicine and a lead author of the study.

Researchers from the academy's Center for Urban Epidemiologic Studies randomly selected just over a thousand people and interviewed them by phone. They found that 7.5 per cent of people living in Manhattan suffered from posttraumatic stress disorder (67,000 people), while 9.7 per cent (87,000 people) reported symptoms of depression.

As the experts had predicted, those people who lived closest to the World Trade Center reported the highest rates of PTSD. In the immediate area, some 20 per cent of New Yorkers reported symptoms like nightmares, anxiety, and outbursts of anger.

"This study provides us with an estimate of psychological consequences in the general population soon after a significant disaster. This will be particularly important for future disaster planning in densely populated urban areas," said Dr. Galea.

Hopefully, such planning will rarely be put to the test.

ROD ALBRECHT
Living in Denial

I grew up across the United States and Canada. My father managed pro football teams. My dad was in football, my mom was in fashion; following the trends of testosterone was the nature of my life.

In the early 1970s, like any pre-teenaged boy, I started . . . I guess you'd call it experimenting. At the time, it was just one more thing you didn't tell your parents about. But in 1972, and I remember it clearly, in 1972, in the fall, I was thirteen at the time, I was sitting on the steps of a friend's house, and for the first time I heard the word "fag." His brother used it, and I had no idea what he was talking about. And I asked, "What's that?" And he told me. Something about "That's guys who do things with guys." And my heart stopped. Just absolutely stopped dead in its tracks. I was suddenly being told that there was this aspect of my life that was beyond inappropriate, that was beyond something you didn't tell your parents. My blood went cold.

Because my dad managed teams in the CFL and NFL, I'd been around naked men my whole life. By ten years old, it wasn't a matter of physical attraction, but no question there was a definite emotional bond. I remember idolizing some of the guys that I knew. I must have led a tremendously sheltered life in the 1960s, because I had no idea that I was different. I remember somebody telling me, "You just never turn the 'girls have cooties' thing off."

When you're growing up, you know the difference between right and wrong, good and bad. And then there's this third category that is, like, nuclear bad. And I don't know if it was intuition or what, but when Robbie said "fag" and explained it to me in the voice of a thirteen-year-old, I knew right then that I was doing something that was nuclear bad. It's not like it opened a Pandora's box of emotions. It was more like it shut the box tight. I knew I was in huge trouble. At twelve or thirteen or fourteen, I don't think you really "show," as the expression might go. And I knew from that moment on that I wasn't ever going to, either.

We moved to Boston shortly after that. And in Boston I fell in love; there was no getting around the issue. I met somebody who was just a really nice person. And for the first time in my life I both fell in love and realized that I was broken. That there was something seriously wrong. And there was no question that it was going to cause me a tremendous amount of anxiety and a tremendous amount of pain.

I was tremendously high-strung. As time went by, I started doing drugs. I think I had an early understanding of the whole kids/Ritalin thing, because I used to do a lot of amphetamines in high school because they'd calm me down. I was also becoming acutely aware of the fact that if I got caught with a guy, it could be really bad for the family. And I was at spring training camp for the New England Patriots in 1973, and for all intents and purposes, I got caught. In the act.

Now it was out – and I was whisked away. My father was going on a scouting trip, and there was no rescheduling it. So they just added me, got me a plane ticket, and off I went. And the only thing I remember about the whole thing is coming home. I remember the limousine pulling into the driveway and my mother was at the living-room window. And when we got into the house she was nowhere to be found. My father came downstairs to my bedroom and said, "Your mother took one look at you and she's in the bathroom throwing up."

I remember my father saying to me when I was caught, "Are you queer?" And I said nothing, really. And he said, "Well, have you ever had any touch-feely thing happen with girls?" And I said, "Yes." And he said, "Oh, thank God, you're bisexual." I'm not going to say my father was tremendously cool about it, but he wasn't bad.

But now it was like, "We will find the pill, we will find the therapy, we will find the whatever that is going to change this, that is going to make this better." I actually think they were far too frightened of anybody finding out to pursue anything.

I felt tremendously cut off. In fact, as soon as Robbie said "fag" in '72, I was cut off. And it just kept getting worse as I got older. And when I realized that I was cut off from the last possible place in the world where I might belong, it was too much. So I did finally follow the unfortunate option of a young gay teenager, and I tried to kill myself. I went down to Miami to spend a couple of days in the world that I could never permanently belong to. And I did it, knowing full well that the end of the weekend would mean that I would have to overdose and die. And I had an amazing time. I had the best time of my life. I think that made it easier to take the pills at the end. At the end of it, it was a huge relief. There was no more anxiety, there was no more paranoia.

My suicide attempt was not discussed in the hospital; it was not discussed when I got out of the hospital. I was given no diagnosis, no medication, no anything. I had been put in the hospital, the damage to the hotel door was paid off (the paramedics had to break it open), and

I was left there until they could get me back to Toronto. *"And if we ever hear of this discussed outside of the house, you can be assured . . . You will not do this to the family. . ."*

I can honestly say that in twenty years of being around football – my dad managed CFL and NFL teams – I think I met three gay players. And then there were maybe two books by players whose careers and lives had been completely ruined by the revelation of their preferences. And I thought, opening the book, "Good for you." And by the end of the book, I'm going, "You're an idiot! You could've just kept your mouth shut and moved on."

As a cover, I was maintaining relationships with girls. And it was . . . I think "pathetic" really best describes it. It was just a matter of this desperate need for companionship above the level of friends. And of course, when you get out of high school, you start living with them – and swearing devoutly that I would never physically betray them in the course of the relationship. Instead, I'd find other faults in her that I could focus on in order to bring the relationship to a point where I could terminate it, or give her the luxury of terminating it.

By the time I was twenty, I was sure that I'd never make it to twenty-one. I thought moving into another industry would change my life, and it didn't. I went to work in the Canadian entertainment industry, and it was not particularly different from football. I remember an artist whose career was infamous, a Canadian artist who was very well-known in the history of rock and roll. He was tremendously well-known because he was associated with so many artists internationally that had become stars. And I remember somebody saying, "But he's a fag. That's why he never made it." And it's, "Oh great – I've made the jump from football to music, and all they've done is take off the equipment."

I hid every single emotional concern behind drugs, behind drinking, behind going out with women, and then behind having relations with men in the worst possible conditions. I had affairs with guys, I even lived with a guy at one point. You develop more than one life. You develop more than two lives. You develop three or four. You really do. Because there's the life that the rest of the world owns that identifies you. There's the life that you own that identifies you in public. And then there's the life that you live, alone in the dark, in the middle of the night.

Even today, living this way is tremendously common. Ten years ago, 75 per cent of the gay men I met were in the closet. And of them, 75 per cent were married. And I just could not comprehend how they managed to do it.

For myself, there was a lot of substance abuse, there was a lot of physical rows and stuff. You know, picking a fight just to blow off the frustration that was building inside you, particularly since I would continually seem to develop crushes on guys that were not in any way, shape, or form available. And in fact, were so distant that there was no way that I could even broach the subject.

And if you're not comfortable with your sexuality . . . every single time I opened the paper, there was something else troubling. And you really do start to look inside and go, "Is the reverend Falwell right? Are these other individuals who are drawing a line connecting being a gay man and being a pedophile – are they right?" And no, they're not. But the fact that I had to even ask myself that question, I think, is an excellent indication of what your mental health is like when you're trying to conceal so much from so many.

I don't think of myself as a late bloomer, but nine years ago I decided to live openly. I started to develop real, sincere feelings that I had done the worst possible thing in the world to the girl that I was living with – that I had betrayed her in the worst possible way, because I wanted out of the relationship and instead of getting into this whole argument and screaming and the rest of it, I just let the relationship die. And when the relationship ended, I went through a year of absolute guilt about what I did to her, and I don't think that will ever go away.

Life became an endless battle. Not one of combat, but of evasion. I was consumed with guilt and pain. Several misdiagnoses later, a doctor finally hit it on the head: rapid-cycling bipolar affective disorder and histrionic personality disorder. One might have triggered the other, but there is no doubt in my mind, living multiple lives and not knowing what safety or self-respect felt like for so long was, is, and will always be the tree from which the monkeys jumped on my back.

A year of tremendous grief and guilt passed, then I came to terms with it. And then I got this job interview for Fresh Start Cleaning and Maintenance. And I decided that I was going to go to the job interview "out." I didn't know how to put it on my resumé, so I actually fabricated something. There was this gay helpline, and I put down on my resumé that I had already been volunteering for them. So, somewhere in the scheme of everything else, they were going to see that I had volunteered for an organization that one would, most likely, not have volunteered for unless one played with that team.

Coming out was like night and day for my mental health. It was absolutely, bar nothing, night and day. This whole other person, I think he wanted to die as fast as I wanted to bury him. Because I shucked that costume the day I got the job. It was just like, that person's dead. Gone.

Seventy-five per cent of everything that was bad in my life disappeared. I just thought that I could *continue* now. No matter what happened, I knew that I'd never have to hurt anybody again. No matter what happened, I would be able to stop risking and just *do*.

With every independent decision I made about who I really was, it was like all of a sudden, in my late thirties, I was deciding that I was going to live my life, that I knew what I wanted to do with the rest of my life. And that was the late-bloomer part. I had avoided dealing with the issue for thirty-seven years.

And at that point my biggest fear was that I was going to lose what sanity I'd gained. There was so much guilt and resentment for the years that I had lost to denial. And I just decided that I wasn't going to let that overwhelm me. There's a great body of evidence today to show that, particularly for adolescent men, if you have any predisposition to mental illness, stress will pull the trigger. And there's no question that I spent much of my life in pain – a constant, non-stop state of underlying pain. Not depression, not anything else. It was just *pain*. Everything hurt. And sometimes the pain was absolutely so bad I didn't think I'd survive, and sometimes it was so bad it was like a little headache in the back of my head. I'll tell you, I was an unwelcome guest in my own home. If that had not happened, I honestly believe there's probably a much greater chance that I would never have developed mental health issues at all.

You spend so much time trying to convince yourself that sexual orientation is not the centre of your life, that it is not the focus of your life, that it *becomes* the focus of your life by trying to fight it. And as soon as you give up the fight, as soon as you give in to the reality of what it is, it becomes, not a secondary issue in your life, or even a *third* issue in your life. It just falls off the chart. I was happy when I finally did it. Now I've managed to get even higher than that, because I think contentment is two or three steps higher.

Now, you know what? If I meet somebody, I'm going to introduce them to the family at some point.

Rod Albrecht is now the executive director of Fresh Start Cleaning and Maintenance, a psychiatric-survivor-run community economic development business in Toronto. Fresh Start was recently named by Profit *magazine, for the second year in a row, as one of the top 200 growing companies in Canada.*

THE (NOT SO) STRAIGHT GOODS

There's a growing body of evidence that gay, lesbian, bisexual, and transgendered youth are at greater risk for mental health problems and suicide than their heterosexual counterparts.

One of the more interesting studies has been taking place at New Zealand's Christchurch School of Medicine, where researchers have been following the long-term health and development of more than a thousand people who were born in mid-1977. As part of that survey, data was collected on any psychiatric disorders these people suffered between the ages of fourteen and twenty-one years. They were also asked if they'd ever dwelled on suicide or made an attempt.

In 1998, the people in the survey were asked about their sexual orientation. Researchers then crunched the numbers to see if there was any difference in the rates of psychiatric disorders between heterosexuals and non-heterosexuals.

They found that gay, lesbian, and bisexual young people were four times as likely to have experienced major depression, nearly three times as likely to have generalized anxiety disorder, five times as likely to smoke, and more than six times as likely to attempt suicide. A recent study from the University of California concludes that "higher levels of discrimination" may be largely responsible for higher rates of mental disorder in the non-straight population.

COLLEEN McDONAGH
"All the Pieces"*

We are not abnormal, we are products of an abnormal experience.
 – Dr. Richard Krell

In the spring of 1988, I was thirty-two years old, and it seemed like all the pieces were finally coming together. I was married to a good man, and we had an adorable seven-year-old son. We had a nice little home in a picket-fence neighbourhood, lots of friends and acquaintances, and, after years of working my way up, I had just landed my dream job. I was living my version of "normal," and life was pure potential.

I'd come a long way from the chaos of my parents' house for this snapshot of normalcy, but the residue of a nasty childhood still hung on me like a thin layer of grime. The nightmares and bleak memories still intruded every chance they got, the desolate and sometimes deranged telephone calls from my mother, the guilt and sadness that always ensued. But whatever I couldn't overlook I could at least cope with, and I felt like I was winning. I had outmanoeuvred the past, and if life wasn't perfect, it was close enough for me.

---

* A portion of this story was first published in a different form on the *Globe and Mail*'s "Facts & Arguments" page.

And then my mother died.

Grief, if suppressed, can be cumulative. The sorrow for what we don't mourn along the way only builds with each successive loss until there is that one thing that cuts us clean in half. For me that "one thing" was my mother's death. Every page of history I'd ever buried, every demon I'd outrun, they were all there, waiting for me, at her funeral. Grief – both old and new – pounded me from all sides, and I went under, down to fossilized memory, to the place where past trumps present.

I am small again. I see my father, face red, teeth clamped over his tongue, eyes glazed with alcohol and fury. I see his fist drive into my mother's face. I see her blood, I hear her screams, the crack of her tiny frame against the furniture. There is drinking and fighting and yelling and crying in this dark house. And there is never, ever enough – enough money, enough alcohol, enough peace. It is pandemonium. The big sisters try to make it better, and when I am older I will learn how, but for now I hide. I know how to hide without leaving the room: I can shrink deep down inside and look forward to tomorrow.

Tomorrow it might be better. No blood, no bruises. Tomorrow it might stop, and my mother might smile at me and tell me I am good – not her curse from the devil, not a tramp. I could be good and lovable. Tomorrow my grandfather might die and I'd be set free from his bony hands and his hot, foul breath and the back bedroom and the ether. I could tell on him then, again, and this time she wouldn't turn away. This time my mother would save me; she would hold me by the shoulders and still the rocking, catch my head in her hands before I banged it against the wall. Tomorrow everything might be quiet.

It never came. The tomorrow I lived for never really arrived, except for this: my grandfather did die. He was murdered. I don't know who it was that set me free.

The drinking and fighting continued, and my mother slipped further away, perhaps into her own imagined tomorrow. One by one the big sisters moved out, each stepping over and around the unacknowledged elephant in our midst that was our past. We never talked about it. Their demons moved with them, crammed and squirming in dark boxes marked *Do Not Open*. This is what survival looks like.

Then there were three, and in time my mother grew to need me the way I had once needed her. When my turn came to leave, I'm quite sure I broke what was left of her heart. She told me it would kill her if I went away; she said I was all she had left to live for. But I could not stay there. I walked away believing my parents had done the best they could with what they had, with their own flawed histories, their own demons. There had to be forgiveness. This is also what survival looks like.

And now she's gone, and I am consumed by guilt.

I tried. I still went to work every morning, still went through the motions of living, but as a barely there phantom, a low-functioning shadow of my former self. I wandered about in a stupor of flashbacks and tiny voices, stiff and hollow as a mannequin, eyes stinging with the risk of tears. Lead filled my veins, and I craved sleep that wouldn't come. Friends and family began to worry, and in anxious tones they told me how life had to go on, how I needed to pull up my socks and move forward. I already felt like a miserable weakling, and knowing that they thought I had a choice made me all the more ashamed. Gradually, their sympathy and concern were exchanged for puzzlement and irritation; in time, they avoided me altogether.

I couldn't tell them. What was I supposed to say? *It seems I am mourning her life as much as her death. A tear for every ounce she drank, every punch she took, every day she spent alone. I am mourning the past that was and the past that wasn't and the future that can't be. Because every time I close my eyes I see her dead face, because her respirator won't stop hissing in my head, because I should have saved her instead of myself. Because I am haunted, because I am drowning, because it's so dark in here. Because I am losing my mind.*

Finding the right help would become the longest, hardest, and most important journey I would ever make. Finding the wrong help cost me almost everything I had, and it very nearly cost me my life.

Getting there was a random process: knocking on the doors of strangers, unaware of the philosophies and doctrines within, even less aware of what they would mean to the care I received. I acted in desperation. In a frame of mind that did not easily permit rational thought, I tried to make major decisions. Most of them were wrong.

I started seeing a psychopharmacologist, and we were both on new ground. He was winding down a psychoanalytic practice to devote himself to biological therapy; I had virtually no experience with psychiatric medication. I needed to talk. He wanted to prescribe, and he did so with all the vigour of a new recruit. A pageant of pills ensued. Imipramine, nortriptyline. *Switch.* On Nardil I became a little manic; he added perphenazine to slow me down. *Switch.* On Prozac I took to cutting myself with an X-Acto knife; he upped the dosage and added lithium and thyroxine. *Switch.* Mellaril. *Switch.* Tegretol. In the thick of it all, I don't know why, I started to drink. A few months and drugs later, I was behind the Plexiglas walls of a locked ward.

I was hospitalized for almost seven months. Seven months, sixteen shock treatments, two hospitals, and a life altered. The doctors said I would likely have little memory of that time, but they were mistaken. So many things were erased or misplaced in those days of loss and disconnection: how to spell, how to sign my name, the face of my own child as an infant. But I did not forget the hospital, or what followed.

Hell is not underground. It is here, on the sixteenth floor. This is the floor no one talks about, the floor where no one talks. Electroconvulsive therapy and drugs like Haldol and Prozac are the chief residents, and everyone lives by their rules. The trust to communicate does not come easily here; everything you say can and will be used against you at Rounds, and silent agreement is generally recognized as the least damning policy.

When I try to retrace the steps that brought me to this place, I encounter the image of my mother's disfigured face against the backdrop of the intensive care unit where she died of meningitis. I lost her once to the alcoholic haze that claimed her when I was a child; I've lost her yet again, and this new loss brings back the old in all its original anguish. The child that surfaces bears the guilt for a family ripped apart by the malignant cruelty and perversion of the paternal grandfather. I can't remember her sober after I tried to tell her what he did to me.

Each time I reach out for help, my soul is anaesthetized with drugs I cannot tolerate and I slide deeper into the darkness. I have lost the job I worked so hard for, and I have lost my house. My friends are gone, and I am pushing the limits of my marriage. My son needs his mother. I am willing to submit to anything that might pull me from this psychic quicksand, but the electroconvulsive therapy makes me worse, and now my memory is as fragmented for the present as it was for the past. For all their chemical wizardry and advanced technology, the one thing they repeatedly deny me is a compassionate human voice. There is time to be interviewed by researchers and tested by interns, but there is no time to talk.

The doctors have determined my condition is intractable, and they are sending me home with four different drugs, a recommendation for maintenance ECT, and the prognosis that I will be hospitalized, repeatedly, for the rest of my life. They used to tell me I was depressed, but under their guidance I have progressed through the psychiatric ranks to "rapid-cycling bipolar affective disorder." The labels are unimportant to me now; all I hear them saying is that I am crazy.

I am going back to the care of the doctor who guided me down the road to this hell because I haven't the presence of mind to go elsewhere. He is the acme of modern biological psychiatry: the brusque little man with the seven-minute appointments; the one who dogmatically and exclusively equates human suffering with chemical malfunction; the one who tells me there is no point in beginning psychotherapy, who armed me with more than 500 pills from failed treatments, pills that call to me from the cabinet with the promise they can end the waking nightmare that has become my life.

The attempt I make to end my life will instead mark its beginning. I am taken to a different place, where the assault against my drug-weary body is stopped and I am unmedicated for the first time in almost two years. I see that I am battered and more than metaphorically crippled, but at least I can see.

My days are punctuated now by the reassuring voice of the gifted therapist who has shown me that the only way out of the dark is to examine it in all its blackness. I am safe here; there are no locked wards, no drugged isolation. The only tools are the human mind and spirit, and a commitment to confront the demons. There is support when I stumble, and wordless celebration in each small victory. I am not crazy, only wounded, and I am alive to heal the wounds because of psychotherapy. Words, my words, can save me.

Fourteen years have passed since my mother died, twelve years since the hospital. I never did go back like they said I would. I stayed in therapy for more than three years, working with the same doctor, sometimes four and five times a week, until he moved away. I used to think he'd saved my life. Now I know he did more than that: he taught me how to save my own.

There have been dark times over the years, and perhaps there always will be. When despair comes, I grit my teeth and let it hurt and try to understand. When it seemed I needed more help, I went back to what I know is right for me, and lately I've returned to psychotherapy. It's different now: this time it is about living, not about surviving. There is no life or death in the balance, but there is more to learn, more light to be had, more peace, and I have earned it. I am in good hands again.

I am not against medication. What I am opposed to is this: a biological mindset that prescribes without listening, the practice of declaring the human condition a disease. Sometimes the heart of sickness is a festering story. That story needs be told, and it needs to be heard.

I have changed. There is no going back to the earlier days of "pure potential," and I'm not sorry now. Those days were built on the backs of ghosts and shadows; they were my house of cards, waiting for the wind to blow.

I am so fortunate. I lived, and I did not lose my husband or my son. This is what matters. We did not recover what was lost all those years ago, but we have rebuilt a life, and it's a good life. I think it will be a better life. The pieces continue to come together.

Colleen McDonagh is pursuing a writing career in Toronto.

PAUSE FOR THOUGHT

"Severe trauma in childhood may have enduring effects into adulthood. . . . Past trauma includes sexual and physical abuse, and parental death, divorce, psychopathology, and substance abuse." (U.S. Surgeon General).

SICK DAYS

- Canadians spent a total of 8.7 million days in hospital for mental disorders in 1998/99. That number has been dropping steadily since the 1970s with the shift to community care and outpatient treatment, along with improvements in medications. It's also almost 2 million fewer days than in 1997/98.
- How long do people stay in hospital, on average?
  - For all causes (cancer, heart disease, surgery, etc.), the average is 8.6 days.
  - On psychiatric wards of general hospitals, the average is 22 days.
  - In psychiatric hospitals, the average is 197 days.
- How common are stays in general hospitals versus psychiatric hospitals? Of the 193,869 discharges related to mental disorder:
  - 87 per cent were from general hospitals
  - 13 per cent were from psychiatric hospitals.

All statistics are from the Canadian Institute for Health Information, 1998/99 figures.

ANDY BARRIE
"Let There Be Light"

"Ninety seconds, Andy," says the producer. "Thirty seconds . . ."

As the clock sweeps with unfailing precision toward the end of the 7:00 a.m. national radio newscast, a relaxed-looking man opens a soundproofed door at the CBC's Broadcasting Centre in Toronto. He walks down a ramp and into the studio where, for three hours every morning, he joins people in their kitchens, their bedrooms, their cars, their offices, their minds. He slips a large monaural headphone over his right ear, a casual gesture as second-nature to him as speaking into a microphone in an empty room. When the theme from the news fades out, a melodic tune fades in. The "ON AIR" light glows red. *Cue.*

"Good morning, I'm Andy Barrie. Welcome back to *Metro Morning*."

The voice listeners are hearing was originally an American one. In fact, a much younger version of it was first heard over the loudspeakers in the summer of 1954 at a place called Camp Skylemar in Maine. There, a beaming nine-year-old was given the job of waking the camp every morning by playing a recorded bugle call over the loudspeaker system. He would also, in a voice much higher in tone, tell campers what the weather would be like that day (after stealing the forecast from a real radio station). Today, a faded but treasured photo of that smiling kid – left hand clutching a microphone near a stack of now-antique records – graces Barrie's very cluttered desk.

Since 1995, Andy Barrie has been part of the morning routine for hundreds of thousands of CBC Radio listeners in and around Toronto. From 6:00 a.m. until 9:00, he's the guy with the knack for asking the question the listener wants answered – whether the topic is serious political discourse or just plain fun. Barrie, along with his producers, serve up news, current affairs, and entertainment five mornings a week. It can be quite an eclectic mix: on this day, they've got a trio that plays traditional Greek folk music performing live in the studio, plus a quirky interview lined up for the final hour.

"We also have, later this morning, a conversation with a woman in Hamilton who found $10,000 on the sidewalk," Barrie teases his audience. (She's a karaoke hostess who found the money in a deposit bag outside a bank machine. After consulting with her parents, she returned it to the grateful bank, which promptly approved her application for a car loan.)

His mellifluous style – which sounds more like a conversation than "announcing" – evolved over more than three decades behind the microphone. After leaving the United States as a conscientious objector to the Vietnam War, he started at CJAD in Montreal in 1970. Barrie eventually settled at the Toronto station that pioneered news and talk radio in this country: CFRB.

There, in the early 1980s, he conducted a fortuitous interview. It was with psychiatrist and author Dr. David Burns, who was then promoting his book *Feeling Good: The New Mood Therapy*. The author helped pioneer something known as "cognitive behavioural therapy," a technique some people successfully use to manage mood and stave off depression.

The night before, Barrie was having a closer look at the work in order to prepare for the interview. It was the first book he'd ever read on depression, and he found the topic fascinating. He was also intrigued by a speedy diagnostic tool it contained, something called the Beck Depression Inventory (BDI). It works by asking the participant twenty-one questions about mood, self-esteem, and behaviour. The subject is asked to rate themselves on a sliding scale of zero to three for each question. For example, "zero" might mean you're never teary, while "three" might indicate you weep frequently.

After answering all the questions, you add up the total. A high score, anything from thirty to sixty-three, means there's a pretty good chance you're suffering from a severe depression. (An unusually low score, by contrast, might mean that you're actually hiding a mood problem; that you're "faking" feeling good.)

"I took this test, and I remember scoring somewhere between 'just fine' and 'a little bit moody,'" says Barrie, the late-afternoon sun spilling into the living room of his Toronto residence. He also remembers, vividly, wondering how *anyone* could possibly feel so terrible that they scored in the higher ranks of the scale. How could a person even function if they felt that awful? It was simply beyond his range of experience. Or at least it was then.

"Fast forward. It's two years later, 1985, and I start feeling, out of nowhere, awful. And I can tell this is *unusually* awful. This is not crummy, this is amazingly bad. And I got this book down, and I took the test again. And damned if I didn't register up there in the stratosphere, where I couldn't believe anybody could breathe air the first time I'd read it."

What had happened? For the life of him, Barrie didn't know. It wasn't as if there'd been a catastrophic event in the past few weeks or months. There'd been no recent death, no undue pressures on the job, no specific catalyst he could pinpoint. It was as if some stranger had surreptitiously slipped a very dark helmet, complete with opaque visor, over his head. Quite simply, quite suddenly, quite inexplicably, Andy Barrie felt like shit. It was, to him, a mystery.

By sheer coincidence, he knew precisely where to go. He was on the board of the Clarke Institute of Psychiatry at the time, and he simply told one of the psychiatrists that he thought he was depressed. Barrie, then forty, was referred to another psychiatrist at a different hospital. He went for three separate visits, the physician exercising caution before rendering a diagnosis. After seeing the consistency of symptoms, he concurred with the results of the BDI: Andy Barrie was clinically depressed.

At the time, there were three main types of medication for treating depression, and different people seemed to respond to the drugs in very different ways. The psychiatrist told Andy the only way to find the best match was to try each med for a time to see what, if anything, worked. He also recommended that they combine the pills with some talk therapy to see if there were some underlying causes for the depression.

"And so we talked," Barrie says. "Certainly, nothing at the time was an obvious trigger. I had not been consciously walking around in any way whatsoever feeling bad about anything. So when you get beyond that, you're getting into a kind of psychiatry that I don't really believe in very deeply, that Freudian psychology in suppressed this and suppressed that."

They tried the first drug and waited several weeks while continuing with talk therapy. Nothing. Barrie switched over to the second antidepressant and waited – hoping each day as he awoke that his internal barometer would rise a notch. Still nothing. By the time they started on the third and final medication, Barrie was getting scared. Yes, he was still managing to go to work every day, still managing to "perform" and get through his on-air shift. But the gulf between the person Barrie was pretending to be when that red light was on and the person who walked out of that studio was widening.

"I was thinking, 'I've got one foot on the dock and one on the boat. Sooner or later, I'm going to fall in the water. How long can I make this last?'"

That balancing act was becoming increasingly precarious. In addition to the effects of the depression itself, Barrie was becoming sick with worry. He still tried to get out, see movies, do normal things, but they often served only to emphasize that he was unwell. He went to see the latest Woody Allen flick, something that would normally leave him with aftershocks of laughter following each punchline. This time, however, he'd chuckle flatly for about a microsecond, followed by . . . zero. An utter and complete absence of anything.

"From inside a brain that was used to the echo of pleasure, it was really weird not hearing it," he explains, searching for the precise analogy. "Like walking into a gymnasium and shouting your name and nothing comes back."

During the eternal wait for the meds to work, Barrie took some solace in reading about others who had successfully recovered from depression. His wife went to the library and returned with *A Season in Hell*, written by Percy Knauth, the former editor of *LOOK* magazine. It gave Barrie hope.

"It was wonderfully comforting . . . amazing to hear someone describing even worse symptoms than I had, who was talking about this from the other side. He described, in his case, how one day it was as if someone had walked over to the light and turned it back on again."

The comfort, however, was tinged with growing concern. It had now been three months since the curtain first descended, and there hadn't been a single change that Barrie could point to as progress. Miraculously, he was still managing to hold it together on-air (partly, he thinks, due to his acting skills). But there were moments when he simply could not mask the distaste he had for the world he found himself trapped in. He recalls one meeting at the radio station where a colleague interpreted the broadcaster's dark mood as personal disdain. "And the guy who was running the meeting snapped at me: 'Do you have a problem with that?' I didn't even know what he was talking about; I was in my own private world. But I was obviously looking the way someone looks who really loathes the idea he's just heard." Barrie later apologized privately, explaining that he'd been "a million miles away." But then, in 1985, on the advice of his doctor, he told no one at the workplace that he was suffering from depression.

As the weeks dragged on, Barrie still managed to cling to the knowledge that, at least in theory, the depression would end, that the light would return. Perhaps, like the book he took solace in, relief would come suddenly.

Eventually, mercifully, that is precisely what happened. Although he'd been treading black water for three months, the transformation occurred literally overnight. "That's what happened. The next morning I woke up, and it was like black and white turned to Technicolor again. I was fine, and I knew that instantly. I didn't feel elevated . . . I didn't feel hyper. I felt great in the sense of revived, the way you do when you get over the flu. I just felt like me again."

For Barrie, the contrast was so sudden he was left shaking his head in detached wonder. It reminded him of photos he'd seen in books of children who, after receiving insulin, went from near-skeletal figures to being the picture of health. "The pure physicality, the mechanicalness of my recovery astounded me."

Once he felt better, he stopped taking the pills, which seems to be what many people do, whether it's antidepressants or antibiotics. Except, about eight months later, he felt he was starting to dip. Not *slide*, exactly, but his early warning system went off and he phoned another psychiatrist he knew. A leading researcher, she said the best evidence showed that some people who've been successfully treated need to remain on a maintenance dose or risk relapse. She suggested Barrie consider it. He didn't need much convincing; he's taken a small dose of antidepressant once a day ever since, and says he's enjoyed the normal range of moods. He also knows that, relatively speaking, he was fortunate.

"I studied linguistics for a while in university, and one of the things you learn in linguistic philosophy is you can't describe pain; there's no way to describe pain. It's a certain kind of first-person statement which is basically incommunicable . . . it's too subjective.

"I know people, certainly, who cannot get out of bed [while depressed]. I've heard these stories; they're paralyzed. That wasn't me. It may have been that my case was not as severe as others might be."

But it was bad enough. So bad, it led Barrie to wonder, at considerable depth, what caused his depressive episode. For that matter, what caused *any* mental illness. More than once, he has thought back to an interview he conducted in 1970. It was with a Canadian researcher who had described compounds in the urine of LSD users similar to compounds found in the urine of people with schizophrenia.

"That was the first clue they had that schizophrenia might be organic. This was revolutionary news," he recalls. "Up until that moment, and for a few years thereafter, the absolute, accepted orthodox view was that schizophrenia was caused by so-called schizophrenogenic mothers [in other words, bad parenting] and the first thing you did with a patient with schizophrenia was get him out of the family."

Barrie found the interview so fascinating, the research so groundbreaking, that he describes it as a "formative experience" of his journalistic and broadcasting career. It was also something of a catalyst for his enduring interest in mental illness and mental health, including that complex and still-debated question: What *causes* this stuff to happen? What, if anything, was behind Barrie's own depressive episode?

Looking back with greater insight now, he thinks there may indeed have been some things going on in his life that contributed to what happened. Yet he knows those events weren't big enough to explain the dramatic and sickening plunge in mood. He also knows those same events would not necessarily have triggered an episode in the next person. So, what happened?

Andy Barrie thinks he has the solution. And he's now read enough, interviewed enough, reflected enough, knows enough, that he's pretty comfortable with the answer: It just *happened*.

"Because I do believe that these things are physical; our brain is an organ. Then the mystery of what triggers mental illness is the same mystery as what triggers all the other biochemical events in the body that make a person cancerous, or diabetic, or get multiple sclerosis, and we could go on and on. It's a trigger."

Barrie believes we have to accept that triggers are biochemical mysteries that – one day – will be unravelled. And we have to view the brain, he says, as another organ. Yes, more complex, but an organ nonetheless.

"The only reason we expect to understand mental illness better goes back to that mind/body dualism. We think there has to have been something on our mind, since the organ that is affected is the brain. 'What did you have on your brain then?' And it's a fair question, I guess, for psychiatrists to ask. But again, we don't usually say to someone who gets cancer, 'What was going on in your life, then?' You don't say to someone with multiple sclerosis, 'What did you have on your neural trunk?' You just say, 'It happened.' So I'm prepared to believe it's a mystery."

As he finishes his story, the late April sun begins to dip sluggishly behind Toronto's angles of brick and steel and glass. Slowly, the colour fades from Barrie's living room. Paintings start losing their hues; book spines drain to variations of grey.

It has been a subtle process, this sinking of the sun. But as the clock strikes 8:00 p.m., it is suddenly apparent that the entire living room, so bright and welcoming just two hours ago, has become monochromatic and textureless. Barrie has his back to the window, and soon even his expressions are difficult to make out.

And then, noticing the change himself, Andy Barrie gets up, takes a few steps, and turns on a light.

DEPRESSION

- Mood disorders affect about 340 million people worldwide at any given time (World Health Organization).

- An estimated 7.1 per cent of the U.S. population has a mood disorder (including unipolar depression, bipolar disorder, and dysthymia) in any given year (U.S. Surgeon General).

- In the year 2000, Canadians made 7,842,000 visits to doctors' offices for depressive disorders — the second-most-common reason after hypertension. That's a 10-per-cent increase over 1999 (IMS Health).

- Depression and distress cost Canadians at least $14.4 billion per year in treatment, medication, lost productivity, and premature death (Health Canada, 1998 estimate).

- Approximately 80 per cent of people with depression respond very positively to treatment (National Institute of Mental Health, U.S.).

SANDY NAIMAN
"Lovesickness"

Words can make you crazy.

Take the word "special." It's like the word "sex." As a kid, I looked up "sex" in the dictionary because it seemed to have many loaded meanings, judging by the cheap magazines Uncle Harry shipped up to the cottage in used brown paper grocery bags. They always showed people naked, eyes blackened out, and with women's nipples and pubic hair and men's penises hidden beneath inky black patches, too. They blackened your fingers. "Sex" screamed from headlines everywhere, but the dictionary definition always differentiated by gender – male versus female. What was all the brouhaha about that? It was the same with the word "special." Sometimes an adult would look down at me and say, "You're special." I never understood why. I certainly didn't feel special, so I'd retreat to the dictionary and look it up. There are fourteen definitions of the word "special." It can mean "individual" and "peculiar" and "distinct" and "different," even "extraordinary." I knew I wasn't extraordinary, because, from the time I was twelve, I had to go to a psychiatrist every week because I was histrionic, another word I had to look up. According to some of my so-called friends, going to a psychiatrist meant I was "crazy," "loony," "nuts," "weird," "bananas," and "mental," all nasty words which can also mean "peculiar" and "distinct" and "different" – none of which I wanted to be in 1960.

As far as my mother was concerned, needing to go to a psychiatrist was like having a broken leg. "When you have a broken leg, you go to a doctor who puts a cast on it so it can heal and get better," she used to say when I complained about how no one I knew went to a psychiatrist and how strange it was to my friends. "It's the same with your mind. If you have a problem with your mind, if your mind isn't well, you go to a psychiatrist who helps it heal. A psychiatrist is a doctor for your mind."

No matter what anybody said, I knew something was very wrong with me. It wasn't constant, but when it happened, when I had what they used to call "a nervous breakdown," I always obsessed about words and dictionaries and writing. Once, for no reason, I was so anxious, I couldn't sleep. But I didn't need to sleep, did I? I was above sleep. What a waste of time sleep was. I would sit in my room at night and write, and when I closed my eyes, all I saw was a huge blackboard with words in white chalk written all over it. I sat up for hours, looking them up in the dictionary and typing the brilliant ideas that were flying inside my head so I wouldn't lose them. I had to record my wondrous ideas, ideas that I read months later and couldn't understand because they were gibberish. Once, while I was in this nervous nocturnal writing mode, something in my mind switched, and instead of reading the dictionary, I started ripping out its pages, beginning at the As, destroying the words that were colliding inside my head. The dictionary was suddenly my enemy; it was evil in my mind, words were the root of my sleeplessness. I had to destroy words. Even when my mother rushed into my room, stopped my ripping, and rescued the huge *Random House Dictionary of the English Language* that she'd given me for my sixteenth birthday, I didn't see how strange my behaviour was.

The next morning, following several muted telephone calls, my mother told me I had to go to the Clarke Institute of Psychiatry. Again. I watched as she packed what I'd need – only nightgowns, toiletries, slippers, a bathrobe. She drove me there, encouraging as always, positive as always, saying that soon I would feel much better, soon I would be able to sleep, soon I would come home. Soon was never soon enough.

After she left me there, alone on the eighth floor, once again, they took away my clothes and locked them up. They asked me to count backwards in sevens from 100 and other pointless questions. They gave me drugs, and sometimes electroconvulsive shock treatments, and eventually I slept. But it was long, lonely months until I could go home again. Nobody ever visited me there, except my mother.

At eighteen, they hadn't yet diagnosed me with manic depression. I was still, according to the psychiatrists, "catatonic" and "schizophrenic," two of the most frightening words of all. There were years of psychiatrists and hospitalizations and drugs and shock treatments. Once, for 24 hours, they even put me into restraints, the most horrifying experience of my life. They put my wrists and ankles into padded leather belts equipped with metal clips that were hooked onto the metal hospital bedposts. They left me there like that, with a bedpan beneath me in case I had to pee or shit. Nothing, nothing was ever as demoralizing and barbaric as that. Nothing. I've never forgotten the feeling of helplessness and the pain of twisting my arms and legs, trying to free myself. Even the shock treatments, which left me with splitting headaches, were innocent compared to the agony of that one night I spent in restraints.

Finally, they found the correct words to describe accurately what was wrong with me. "You have a unipolar mood disorder with a vulnerability to mania."

It's rare, my brand of mood disorder. Most people go up and down. They fly high and fall hard, but I've never experienced that fall – only the delusions, the grandeur, and the speeding thoughts. Once, I drove down to the newsroom at four a.m. It seemed, and I remember the feeling vividly, as if my car was expanding beneath me as I drove. It felt like it was a flying carpet on automatic pilot just a few feet above

Bayview Avenue. Firmly convinced I was the publisher of the *Toronto Sun*, where I'd worked for years, I was determined to breeze into the newsroom and input into my computer my master plan for a total redesign of the paper's personnel – who would be hired, fired, and re-assigned new posts. I gave myself a plum position as a "wild card" columnist to write about any subject of interest whenever I wished, in my own office with a window facing onto King Street.

On another night, I drove down to the *Sun*, always a safe refuge, my second home, and I went upstairs to my second-floor desk. A security man found me there and made no fuss but recognized that I wasn't myself. Instead of trying to eject me, he kindly brought me tea and toast to soothe what he could see was my extreme agitation. He took care of me, as the *Sun* always has, from every quarter. When I drove back to my apartment, I phoned my mother and she knew as she always did, from just the sound of my voice, that I was flying without the aid of any magic carpet and needed to be hospitalized.

Today, the first ninety-nine pages of my *Random House Dictionary of the English Language* – all the As until the word "author" – remain tattered and torn, a tangible reminder of my temporary but recurrent bouts of insanity, psychosis, mania.

Words still make me crazy, as they do any perfectionist-writer, I tell myself. As a journalist, a feature writer for twenty-five years with the *Sun*, I'm never satisfied with my stories, my writing, and my words. They're never good enough. I'm never good enough. That's what Dr. Bob is always bugging me about.

When I lie in bed in the morning in the twilight of wakefulness, fresh from a dream, while Marty, the man who actually had the nerve to marry me, is downstairs making coffee, for a few seconds I feel normal. It's fleeting, that feeling of normalcy, that feeling of oneness with the rest of the world. I actually feel loved for the first time in my fifty-three years until I remind myself not to forget to take my medication and that if I don't, in the world out there I can still become, quite literally, crazy. The last time I was hospitalized was when I first met Marty and I realized he was actually real and his feelings for me were real, as he expressed them with his words, his kisses, and his touching. This was an astounding revelation. This couldn't be, but it was and it propelled me into the heavens, it was so remarkable.

Those heavens, however, were perilous, because nobody really believed me. Not even my mother. Everyone thought Marty was a fantasy, like all the others, and tried to convince me that I was high, which drove me even crazier. In the past, every time I got high and was hospitalized, which was nineteen or twenty times, there's been some strange mental sexual connection. And some man. I never had sex – though that would have been lovely – I just fantasized about sex and a man, some man who may have treated me kindly or upon whom I had a crush. In my mind, somehow, he and his kindnesses metamorphosed into love, or what I imagined love to be, since I'd never been there before. Too many times, because I got high on some fantasized love, some imagined passion robbed me of sleep and fuelled my wild and wicked obsession with words. I'd be taken to the mental ward and promised that I'd feel better soon, but too many times "soon" translated into months. Not soon, as I'd imagined soon to be. It's never soon, when you're on the inside, where it's a major effort to make a telephone call (there was only a pay telephone on the ward, and I never had the right change). No one visits or sends cards or even wants to know where you are when you're in a mental ward. And no one – positively no one – loves you, except your mother.

For some reason I only now understand, when I was hospitalized doctors began to fill the places of those fantasy men, whom I imagined loved me. If I couldn't sleep – and insomnia plagued me when I was hospitalized – I imagined a doctor was going to come in the middle of the night and rescue me and take me away. Doctors were my knights, but instead of wearing shining armour, they wore white coats; and instead of carrying lances and shields, they carried metal clipboards and ballpoint pens. They listened carefully and seemed compassionate, but they never rescued me, especially in the middle of the night. No one ever did, but this fantasy was almost as comforting as the fantasy that there was a man out there somewhere, who loved me passionately and desperately wanted to make love to me.

For more than thirty years, this fantasy played tricks with my mind. I'm not alone. Once, when researching a story on the biology of love, a professor of medieval English literature in Los Angeles told me of a collection of sixteenth-century monographs of women who, like me, fantasized about men who loved them or whom they believed they loved. It seems their fantasies drove them mad. At that time, the name given this curious malady was "lovesickness." But what psychiatrist would believe you if you told him you had medieval lovesickness? He'd just think you were crazy. Except Dr. Bob. He confirmed this diagnosis for me.

There's a reason for my lovesickness. The first time I was hospitalized, I was not high. I was fourteen years old, and a child psychiatrist wanted me there "for observation." I was put into a single room in an old, dilapidated ward. I couldn't sleep and the nurses were nasty. It was fourteen years later that I remembered what happened to me in that ward, and the memory still haunts me.

It was evening, after dinner, and there was nothing to do. This was 1962 and psychiatry wards weren't the most well-equipped places. Charitable donations tended to go to more high-profile illnesses. Mental illness wasn't, and still isn't, one of them. It's too stigmatized.

My room had only a bed, a small dresser, an old wooden chair with a green vinyl seat cover, ugly torn curtains, and grey-green walls with spider cracks running along the ceiling. I couldn't sleep, so the nurse gave me something that made me drowsy. But it didn't make me sleep, so I lay awake, not quite alert. A doctor, a man wearing a white coat, came into my room and started asking me why I wasn't sleeping. He wasn't familiar, and I can't remember if he was wearing a name tag on his lapel like the other doctors. But he seemed nice and took the time to talk to me, more time than any of the nurses. He stepped closer to my bed. I was lying down, looking at the ceiling and imagining where the spiders were, when he reached over to touch my shoulder. His hand was warm and he said he could help me sleep. My mind seemed clouded, but I didn't resist. He spoke softly. Slowly, he reached beneath the covers and slipped his hand down, down between my legs, where he started to touch me, to feel me with his fingers. It felt good, and bad.

Nice, but not right. But I didn't have the energy to stop or fight. He was doing things with his fingers that felt so good and I was tingling. I don't remember how long he did it, just how good it felt, how warm. Like nothing I'd ever felt before. And then, somehow, I slept.

That man, a doctor as far as I could tell, had made me feel so good, so good. But it wasn't right, somehow. That's why I forgot about it for years. And when the memory surfaced, things began to make sense. I confided in my mother, and together we could begin to see why I was the way I was. Until I was fourteen, I was always a normal weight, but within six months of being on that hospital ward, I gained fifty pounds. Food couldn't satisfy my hunger, and the fat fleshing me out shielded me from men who might try to hurt me or invade me or assault me. For years, my weight yo-yoed. And still does. Food was and is an issue. Food medicates. Dulls your pain. Men intimidated me, though I never consciously understood why.

One day, not long after I shared this memory with my mother, she came home from her Tuesday evening session of volunteering at the Toronto Distress Centre looking drawn and tired. She told me about a call she'd taken from a distraught woman whose father had recently died. This woman was hysterical because finally she could confess to a horror she'd secretly harboured for years. Her father had been an orderly at the same hospital I'd stayed at in 1962. He had sexually abused her for years, as a child, and she was desperately afraid he may have sexually abused other young women at the hospital. It wasn't difficult to calculate the overlap in years, and to assume, probably correctly, that the man, the so-called doctor, who had assaulted me when I was so innocent, was this woman's father. Now he was dead, but his residual damage lives on. No wonder I've confused doctors with romance and rescue.

When Marty and I met, something peculiar happened. I felt completely free to be myself, and he was such a joy. All those old fears seemed to evaporate into the humid July air and everything was so easy. That was almost three years ago, and even though I had to be hospitalized soon after – my romantic high made me a little hypomanic – he rescued me. He's not a doctor of medicine, but he doctors scripts – he's a respected dramatist and screenwriter. He visited me in the hospital and took me out for romantic dinners and quickies in my apartment. Even my dog, Murphy, liked him. And ever since I've married him, my mother isn't the only one who can tell, just by my voice, if I'm getting high. He can, too.

I am safe and saner than ever.

Journalist Sandy Naiman has written features for the Toronto Sun *since 1977 and is a passionate stigma-buster and vocal advocate for people living with mental illness. Married to writer Martin Lager, she can now add step-mothering to her list of accomplishments.*

MENTAL ILLNESS AND SEXUAL ABUSE

▶ An Ontario survey of ten thousand adults found that 11 per cent of women and 4 per cent of men reported a history of *severe* sexual abuse in childhood.

▶ Childhood physical abuse is associated with anxiety disorders and alcohol abuse in adulthood. In women, it's also associated with major depression and illicit drug abuse. "A history of childhood sexual abuse was also associated with higher rates of all disorders considered in women," say the Canadian authors of a paper published in 2001 in the *American Journal of Psychiatry.* They conclude that "a history of abuse in childhood increases the likelihood of lifetime psychopathology," especially for women.

▶ Sexual and/or physical abuse in childhood is also associated with more reports of self-injury, suicidal ideation, and suicidal behaviour in adulthood.

▶ The U.S. Surgeon General reports that more than 25 per cent of child sexual abuse cases involve a parent or parent substitute.

▶ "The long-term consequences of past childhood sexual abuse are profound, yet vary in expression," reports the U.S. Surgeon General.

―m―

This guy is driving his sporty convertible in the countryside. It's a gorgeous day and he's got the top down.

Unbeknownst to him, however, the lug-nuts are slowly rattling loose on his front left wheel. He feels the steering get wobbly and pulls over just outside the gates of a psychiatric hospital.

The driver gets out and sees that all four lug-nuts have gone. There's nothing holding the wheel on the car, and he can't start driving again or it will fall off. He's scratching his head when a patient, out for a walk in the grounds, sees he is in a quandry.

"Hey!" says the patient. "Why don't you take one lug-nut off each of the other three wheels and bolt your tire on? That'll last until you get to a service station."

The driver's eyes brighten as he realizes his conundrum has been solved. He thanks the patient, but can't help looking surprised that he'd come up with such a clever solution.

"Just because I'm crazy," the patient says with a smile, "doesn't mean I'm stupid."

Variations of this story have been told at countless mental health conferences and in more than a few patient lounges. It is told to illustrate just one of the many false stereotypes people face when they attempt to make a re-entry into the real world after an encounter with illness: the notion that people with a mental illness are somehow stupid, or weak, or defective. Such negative and discriminatory beliefs throw roadblocks into the recovery process.

Yet people do recover. For some, it's as simple as finding the right pill. As we saw with Andy Barrie, there are cases where the medication alone simply clicks and the problem goes away. Many others pursue a combination of meds plus psychotherapy (which generally produces the best results).

But the process of recovery, of moving on, is as individual as the people we've met. Some have pursued alternative therapies that worked for them (we strongly urge anyone on medication to consult with a doctor before considering a different path), others have thrown themselves head-first into advocacy. Those who've experienced isolation and poverty found that, in addition to meds, having meaningful work and social contact were crucial to wellness.

There are, we believe, countless paths to recovery. What works for one person may not work for the next. And while we won't even get into the debate about psychotropic medications, we strongly believe that most people need more than a pill to improve their lives. They need a sense of meaning, of purpose, of life beyond the diagnosis.

We cannot endorse any single treatment option – nor would we – because recovery is about searching. About slowly identifying the road ahead, planning a way to get down that road – perhaps seeing if you can find a good friend who'll join you for that walk.

This chapter is about nine people who all searched before eventually finding nine different paths to recovery. They are stories that inspire us, amuse us, and make us want to celebrate just how diverse and truly remarkable human beings are. Stories that spur us, literally, to stand up and applaud.

They are also people who remind us, a final time, where labels belong: on soup cans.

DEREK WILKEN AND MELANIE GRACE
On Humour

Derek: I never thought I would end up being a comic.

Growing up, I was considered gifted. (Mind you, I was from Saskatchewan!) I skipped Grade 4, was drafted to play Junior A hockey in my teens, and started a business when I was twenty-two. Our company made an insulating cover for oil and gas refinery equipment; with the boom in oil prices, I was soon in charge of a business with more than twenty employees. I was on top of the world. I was married, had two kids, and owned a beautiful, large house on the Bow River in Calgary. But what goes up . . .

Melanie: I got into the comedy business after losing my job, my fiancé, and my mom in the space of about a year. (My fiancé didn't die – he just dumped me six days before the wedding. So I just *wished* him dead!)

I was having problems sleeping, so I would watch David Letterman late at night. The laughter and humour helped me get to sleep, and the next day I had something funny to think and talk about. This meant that I had periods of joy amongst the feelings of angst and was a lot more fun to be with.

I started pondering how I could make my life, and the lives of others, a little lighter and brighter. But I wasn't sure how to do it. I was not a comedian myself . . . a ham maybe, but not a comedian. When I heard that the Calgary office of the Canadian Mental Health Association (CMHA) was forming a committee to develop a mental illness awareness and prevention program for high school students, I thought, "It doesn't sound funny, but it sounds like it would be fun, rewarding, and worthwhile."

I went for an interview, and that's where I met Derek. Derek claims that he fell in love the instant I touched his puffins. For me, it was love, or at least chemistry, at first sight. There was something exciting, even electrifying about him. (I learned later that it's called mental illness.) He was tall, had long, wild-looking grey hair, and was wearing a black

T-shirt with puffins all over it – the elusive (to me), highly sought-after (by me), adorable, fun little bird. Being not quite 5'4", I have always said that good things come in small packages.

I never believed in "destiny" or "fate," but when I found out that he ran a humour therapy program . . . I became a believer!

Derek: I like to say I got into comedy by accident – I was run over by a Volvo, hospitalized, and told I had a mental illness. Then everything fell apart. The joke I use to explain it to people is: Do you know what it's like to be run over by a Volvo? It's bumper-ground-muffler-ground-out. The last thing I saw was a tire with "Goodyear" on it, and I remember thinking, "Probably not *this* year!"

I got into comedy after being diagnosed with bipolar disorder because it seemed to be the only career open to me. I was twenty-seven years old, a recently failed business owner, and for some reason very open about my condition. I was still in denial, and so the cycle would repeat: new job, tell them I was crazy, lose job, go crazy.

I became homeless because I wore out my safety net. Everyone around me was scared of the condition, I couldn't find a job, and trying to live on welfare cheques of $312 per month made having a place impossible. I lived in a warehouse, or outside, or in transit with temporary friends. The street people I used to perform comedy for gave me the nickname "Derelict," and it stuck. I started doing jokes at comedy clubs about being homeless. They went something like this: A friend of mine invited me to come see his new place. I'm a little out of touch with domestic occasions. What do you give to a person who has just moved into a station wagon – air freshener?

Comedy gave me the chance to talk about my pain in a way that was both empowering to me and non-threatening to those I was trying to connect with. If I tell you I have a mental illness, chances are you will want to find the nearest exit. If I make you laugh, you'll still want to run, but you will be smiling as you flee.

I had to learn comedy the hard way. I went to amateur nights at local comedy clubs, offered to perform free in bars, strip clubs, and schools. I had performed over 300 times before I was actually paid, and that was when the guys at the strip club threw loonies at me.

After years of learning the craft of stand-up comedy, I concluded that it was something I could teach others. You know what they say, those who can't . . . teach!

In 1995 the City of Calgary agreed to fund my delusion. In concert with the CMHA, I created a training course and called it the Cheers Project. The purpose was to teach people with a mental illness the skills of stand-up comedy. They could then use the skills onstage at a comedy club and in their lives. It was during this time that I met Melanie. When I told her what I was doing, she became more excited about the concept than I was. She seemed to be on a mission. I was in love.

Melanie: Derek and I both joined the CMHA education committee. After several months, I ended up getting a paid position at CMHA. There was never a dull moment. I was working with people who were depressed, delusional, and suicidal . . . and that was on a good day! I wanted to help them, but felt frustrated working within a so-called "mental health" system that was often not flexible or accommodating enough to meet their needs.

I became increasingly interested in what Derek had to offer, both personally and professionally. The laughter and humour we shared energized me. I wanted to share this source of joy with others.

I was passionate about his project (Derek wasn't too bad either). I offered to be his manager. The fact that I had never managed anyone before didn't bother Derek.

In June 1998, after two years working at CMHA, I took the plunge. I quit my job and began working full-time with Derek to develop, promote, and deliver the Cheers Project. We married that August.

We began delivering presentations and workshops to non-profit organizations and did a lot of work for mental health organizations. Three psychologists did research on our program; they concluded that it improved interpersonal skills, increased confidence and self-esteem, and reduced social isolation, anxiety, and feelings of depression. It also helped people with the ability to cope, manage anger, and empathize with others. Using humour to talk about mental illness also decreased the feeling of stigma while increasing a sense of self-worth. As one mental health participant said, "For the first time, we saw ourselves as unique, creative individuals."

Soon, local and national magazines, radio, newspaper, and TV got wind of what we were doing. Many reporters, columnists, and talk-show hosts thought it was a great "human interest" story. Our name was getting out, and people across the country were calling us. In no time, we were delivering keynotes and workshops across Canada, to everyone from athletes to accountants, panhandlers to professional speakers, evangelists to engineers.

Derek is, however, most proud of our ongoing work with the Calgary Police Service. He delivers a routine to recruits called "The Arresting Benefits of Humour." The goal is to raise awareness and understanding of mental illness and demonstrate how to use humour to communicate and reduce conflict.

Derek: Anyone who is mentally ill and living on the streets sees a side of policing most of us could never imagine. If I caused any of my family members concern, they would take a court order out on me. This would mean I was picked up by the police and taken to a hospital for evaluation. This is not a pleasant task for the police and was usually a painful and humiliating one for me. Any sign of resistance was met with often brutal force. There was only one time that it was easy. The officer came up to me and asked me what I did for a living. I told him I was trying to become a comic. He replied, "Armed with your wit, eh?" For some reason I went easily with that guy.

When I was first asked to do a presentation for the police, I was bitter. As a comic I blew it; instead of using humour to change attitudes, I delivered a lecture. After watching the videotape of my presentation, I thought, "I'd better practise what I preach." I now put everything I have into these sessions. If I can show just one recruit that the best way of approaching a mentally ill person is with a sense of humour, I will have succeeded.

Melanie: In order to teach stand-up, I started as a student of Derek's in a comedy course for the Brain Injury Rehabilitation Centre. All the students, except me, had a brain injury, a mental illness, or both. We met once a week. Derek taught us how to write, tell jokes, and put the jokes together to create a routine. We learned how to project our voices, handle a microphone, and think on our feet.

I was inspired by how creative, enthusiastic, determined, and productive my fellow classmates were. Two of the students had previously been paralyzed and in comas; after their brain injuries, they had to learn to walk and talk again. One had also developed schizophrenia and was incredibly delusional. I was amazed at how they were able to think and speak more clearly when they were focusing on their jokes. It was evident that the course had more than psychological benefits for them.

Working on our routines consumed us. I would sometimes wake Derek at three in the morning to try out a new joke. You become so focused on being funny and finding the funny perspective on your problems, that your problems lose their power over you.

Finally, after six weeks of classes, the night came for us to perform our show. Hundreds of people packed the room. Nothing could prepare me for the feeling of terror before I went on.

Against Derek's recommendation, I went on stage without notes. I had memorized my routine, so I didn't feel I needed them. I ploughed through my material and everything was going relatively smoothly. I don't know how funny I was, but I managed to talk and stay conscious.

Suddenly, my mind went blank! I couldn't think of a thing to say! I panicked. I didn't know what to do. Finally, after what seemed like an eternity, Derek yelled out a cue. Thank God, he knew my routine. Everyone burst out laughing when I said, "Oh yeah," then continued my routine.

Comedy relies on releasing tension. I certainly provided the tension. Good thing Derek provided the release!

When I was done, I felt like I'd climbed Mount Everest. It was the scariest thing I'd ever done in my life, and I had survived. The feeling of power was addictive. I felt like I could do anything after that. That's part of the allure.

Derek: More than any physical, psychological, or humorous benefit, creating the Cheers Project has given me new respect for marriage counsellors. Melanie and I have made a point of injecting "cheer" into our marriage. We often fail, but we never quit. To have fun in life mostly depends on how we interact with those we spend time with. If you are around an individual or group in "ill humour," chances are it will rub off on you. Making light of a problem might encourage the people in your life to despise you, but then you can always use them in your jokes.

If there is one universal "skill" we teach it is that life will deal you blows that you have no way to prepare for. It could be a physical or emotional illness, a death, or just the irrational behaviour of the people around you. If you can *consciously* choose to see these events in the light of humour, not only will you survive, but those around you will have a better chance. We can teach the skills; it's up to everyone individually to use them.

Stand-up comedy is a powerful cathartic experience. I call it "naked skydiving without the sense of security."

Derek and Melanie: One of the first Cheers graduates was Joyce Hunter, a grandmother who struggled each day with manic depression and severe heart and kidney problems. She would come to class straight from her dialysis three times a week. Once, she came to class after having heart surgery. In a radio interview about the Cheers Project, Joyce said this about its therapeutic benefits: "I think it lifts the immersion in self . . . self-pity, self-absorption. It gives you a different slant on your personality." She said that her comedy performance gave her confidence and comfort and that her family had never laughed so hard in their lives.

Joyce Hunter passed away at the age of sixty-seven on June 12, 2001. The minister at the memorial service said that Joyce's greatest wish was to be ordained as a minister but she could not be because of her bipolar disorder; she was, however, able to minister through her work with the Cheers Project.

We show the videotape of Joyce's performance to people across the country. It never fails to educate, entertain, and inspire.

We would like to dedicate our story to Joyce Hunter. People like Joyce make it all worthwhile.

Derek Wilken describes himself as an honorary MD (for Manic-Depression). Noting that one in five people has a mental illness, he is often heard advising people to look around, because "if the four people closest to you seem okay, you may have a problem."

Melanie Grace says the BA after her name means Bipolar Associate (as well as Bachelor of Arts in Psychology). Raised by hippies, she reports that she learned teamwork from her parents. "I cut the grass. They rolled it. I was fourteen before I discovered baggies were for sandwiches."

For more on the Cheers Project, visit their Web site at <www.cheersproject.com>.

HAPPY TALK

▶ We laugh roughly seventeen times on an average day (although children laugh even more often).

▶ Humour has been found to enhance the immune system, release endorphins, relax muscles, and decrease blood pressure.

▶ Twenty seconds of hard belly laughing burns the same number of calories as three minutes on a rowing machine. (Or, as Derek puts it, "more giggling equals less jiggling.")

RONA MAYNARD
On Psychotherapy

Rona Maynard first set foot in a psychotherapist's office when she was nine years old. She was in the third grade and, despite her obvious intelligence, had fared poorly on an aptitude test, leading a teacher to conclude that young Rona must be an underachiever. Soon, she and her mother were making weekly trips to a clinic, Rona coaxed with toys into play therapy while Fredelle Maynard sat in session with the doctor.

Decades later, Rona would return to psychotherapy with more fruitful results. But this was small-town New Hampshire in the 1950s, a time she refers to wryly as "the Dark Ages" of therapy. "My mother . . . talked in circles, by the sound of things, because the fact that her husband was an alcoholic was never addressed. And I played with a very sweet-natured woman who occasionally asked me questions about the toys. The only benefit of this therapy was that I got some undivided attention from my mother, who had to drive me to the clinic and drive me back every week."

Maynard shares this childhood memory while seated in her large corner office on the eighth floor of a sprawling, ultra-modern office/retail complex in Toronto's downtown core. From here, the label of underachiever looks patently absurd. She oversees an editorial staff of twenty-four people who produce, each month, the largest-circulation women's magazine in Canada.

It's early summer now, a busy time at *Chatelaine*. Women of all ages, sizes, and styles of dress – jeans, formal suits, one unlikely black-on-black skirt-over-leggings combo – are working together on the all-important September issue. Maynard herself is dressed loosely in black with a splash of colour from her purple-painted toenails. Her hair is pixie-short and her build is tiny as tiny can be. What stands out most about her, though, is her utter composure. At fifty-three, she has poise down to an enviable art form.

It has not always been so. "I know how it feels to be a real outsider," she assures us. "I know how it feels to have people make fun of you. I was a very strange kid. . . . Kids did terrible things to me. And I have learned from that experience."

Raised in an über-achieving household, Rona and younger sister Joyce were both precocious writers, winning prizes and publishing in national magazines while still in high school. No less was expected of them. Their Canadian-born mother, Fredelle, had a Ph.D. from Radcliffe – this in the 1950s! – and wrote books later in life. Father Max was an English professor who had once been an apprentice of Emily Carr; his landscape paintings can still be found in Canadian art galleries.

"My parents were passionate in their love of the arts and ideas; they were creative people," Maynard says. "They were formidably articulate."

Formidable, too, at keeping painful secrets.

"The alcoholic's family is always a nest of secrets and deceptions," Fredelle wrote in her second memoir, *The Tree of Life*. "Ours was perhaps worse than most."

Joyce later wrote in *her* second memoir, *At Home in the World*, "There are two stories: the way life really is in our family, and the way we make it look to the world." (Joyce is, yes, *that* Joyce Maynard, who wrote a cover story for the *New York Times Magazine* at eighteen, attracting the attentions of fifty-three-old J. D. Salinger and later the outrage of the literary community when she wrote about their tortured relationship.)

The two sisters responded, and struggled, in different ways. Joyce craved attention, and in her teens developed eating disorders. Rona, "remote, almost regal," as Fredelle would describe her, retreated to her books, her guitar, and her collection of mournful Joan Baez records. From the age of nine she lived with her own unnamed affliction: depression. "The whole household revolved around my father's needs, and I was a very, very quiet child," she says. "I internalized everything. My sister was more of an acting-out child, and she got a great deal of attention by being finicky about her food, for example. That was the only way she could get anyone to pay any attention. I didn't discuss the way I felt."

Maynard now believes her father's alcoholism was a form of self-medication; his primary problem, she's quite sure, was a lifelong undiagnosed depression. Young Rona's moods would likewise go undiagnosed for many years. "I certainly did have very prolonged periods, lasting for months, when I was without hope. And I'd say that's depression." At home, she was a door-slammer; at school, she was painfully shy. And in her teens, she was "very very moody. . . . I would drink to get drunk." One line from a Kurt Vonnegut novel stuck with her: " 'Everything is going to get worse and worse, and never get better again.' That was definitely my attitude, on and off, for years. And the bad times would last for months."

Her depression was never so severe that life could not carry on around it. At seventeen, Maynard left home for university; a year later she moved to Toronto; on her twenty-first birthday, she married; and at twenty-two she became a mother. The recurring dips in mood were more like a low-grade fever that leaves you, if not bedridden, then weakened and at times incapable of enjoying anything.

The worst of it came, as is often the case for women, with new motherhood. "I had a crashing depression after Ben was born," she says. "And I didn't know what was wrong with me, why I was feeling this way. Nobody I knew had a baby, so I didn't have anybody I could talk to about this. My friends were bumming around Europe, very carefree, [or] going to graduate school." Maynard, meanwhile, was spending her days alone with her baby in a tiny apartment while her husband was at work. "We hadn't planned the pregnancy," she wrote in a *Chatelaine* article, "and neither of us had ever changed a diaper. Even worse, Benjamin was colicky, and I didn't feel the promised surge of maternal love."

Those first months of motherhood – the sleepless nights, the isolation, and all the incumbent frustrations – would induce the worst depression of her life. Unfortunately, in the 1970s, postpartum depression was not widely recognized; Maynard had no idea why she was struggling. Much of what she was feeling, however, was textbook postpartum depression. "I'm told by people who saw me with Ben that

I could be very tender and playful and loving, and I do remember a little of that. But I'm afraid that a lot of what I remember is just not really being there emotionally, just wishing he would go away. One day, when he was very tiny, just newborn, I remember thinking, 'I'd like to throw my baby out the window.' I wouldn't have actually done it, but I was so unhappy. . . . It terrified me, but you couldn't talk about those things. I thought I must be a pretty hard-hearted, unloving, incompetent mother to have such a thing even cross my mind."

Years later, Rona Maynard learned that she, too, had been a colicky baby, and that Fredelle had lived with some of the same frustrations of new motherhood. But at the time, she says, "I would look at my adorable baby and I would see my own failure."

When Ben was three, Maynard took a full-time editing job, the start of a lifelong career in magazines. Her mood improved, but not for long. "I hid behind a mask of competence," she has written, "meeting every deadline and making fettucine from scratch." Keeping her depression hidden would leave her physically depleted. Colleagues would later say they remembered her most often with a coffee cup in one hand and an Aspirin bottle in the other.

For many years, it had never occurred to her to seek help for her dips in mood. "I thought I was very tough and strong," she says. "'I don't need anybody; I'm very independent. Nobody can help me anyway.'" But in her mid-thirties, Rona Maynard finally took action. Working at home as a freelance writer, "it all started to close in again. I began thinking that I didn't have a reason to live. . . . I remember thinking, 'Well, if all else fails, I have a bathtub and a razor blade.' And this would go through my mind all day long."

She picked up the phone, called a women's clinic, asked to see a therapist. "I decided I would have to get a life." The clinic connected her with a psychiatrist she had once interviewed for a story. "I didn't like her at all. But she was very effective," Maynard says bluntly. "I felt that she was going to raise the bar for me. She had high expectations for me emotionally, and I didn't for myself. . . . I needed someone to convince me that I could aspire to more."

This particular psychiatrist took an unusually cerebral approach. Maynard remembers lectures on Freud and many theoretical discussions. In a *Chatelaine* editorial, she describes their early relationship. "It took her all of half an hour to dismiss my theory on the roots of my despair and assert her own. 'There's going to have to be a reorganization here!' she vowed, as if I were a graduate student whose thesis was going off the rails. Much as I disliked her, I wanted top honours."

Maynard's mood improved rapidly with talk therapy, and without any prescribed medications. "I'd been expecting to get a prescription, but I didn't. . . . My psychiatrist told me they would not be helpful in my case. She said I was suffering from a reactive depression and that, in essence, I had just learned some very unhappy-making ways of looking at my world and myself." Over the next year or so, regular therapy sessions became a kind of escape valve for her feelings. "I started expressing things, instead of keeping them inside. My husband noticed quite rapidly that my behaviour had changed for the better; I was just nicer to be around."

For the first time in her life, she turned to exercise, hitting the running track until her knees gave out. Her energy levels and self-esteem soared. She's since switched to gentler pursuits: walking, yoga, posture work. And it shows in her admirably upright frame – "I find it uncomfortable to slouch" – as well as in the pink sock that sits on her office filing cabinet, stuffed with tennis balls, ready to combat neck pain.

Through therapy, Maynard has learned how to take better care of herself, both physically and emotionally. Now, when she feels an occasional dark mood start to settle in, she knows how to stop it in its tracks. She still takes short "refresher courses" of therapy, targeting a specific goal or issue, whenever she feels it is necessary.

The therapy, the exercise, the long process of making for herself "a life worth living" has imbued in Maynard a new sense of her place in the world. And this is what pleases her most. "To me there is something miraculous about waking up in the morning and looking forward to my day," she says, "and seeing challenges as things to overcome and learn from, not things that could crush me."

Today, Rona Maynard is not remotely interested in the sometimes grim, sometimes angry details of her past depression. She's been healthy for more than fifteen years, and what *does* interest her still is the path out, those individually constructed mazes we must find our own way through. "Depression is exceedingly boring," she declares. "You have to find a way to deal with it, and that's what's interesting."

And that's why the woman who for decades kept secrets can today be found behind the podium at the venerable Ontario Club, speaking to a tony crowd at a fundraiser for a psychiatric research foundation. (She appears at any number of such worthy events.) Not so long ago, the well-heeled ladies and men in tailored suits would not have dared discuss such an unseemly topic at lunch. But here is Rona Maynard, editor of *Chatelaine*, framed by a swath of red velvet curtains, leaning into a microphone as she describes with good humour and fine detail the "terrible taint" of depression. The crowd, sipping coffee, is rapt. She tells them she has decided she hates waste. And that *not* talking about those years would constitute a waste.

So she talks. And she writes, hoping others will see in her story the possibilities that exist within their own.

Maynard once told a *Toronto Star* reporter that, having felt cut off from the world in childhood, writing has become in adulthood "a way of rejoining the human race." And this is perhaps nowhere more true than in her columns about depression. Each time she writes on the subject, offering another piece of her story, grateful letters, e-mail, and phone calls flood in. Readers share their own experiences with her, often never having spoken of them before.

"I know that only good can come of having more open discussions about what depression does to people's lives. Not just the life of the sufferer, but the lives of the people around that person. I've seen this as an employer. I've seen it as a friend."

Despite the bustle beyond her door, Maynard's office, with its lilac-coloured walls, has the feel of a quiet oasis. On one of those walls, she's hung a small chalk drawing of purple spring flowers in a field of tall grass. "That was done for me by a reader who has suffered from depression," she explains, "a young man, and he wanted to thank me for raising this subject in my editorial. He said that my words gave him hope, and here's a symbol of hope; it's a picture of spring flowers."

She keeps the picture by the window overlooking Bay Street, just above her blue iMac. She sees it there each time she pauses, for a moment, from her work.

MORE THAN BABY BLUES

▶ Depression is perhaps the best known postpartum disorder, but new mothers may also experience postpartum anxiety, mania, OCD, and psychosis. Combined, these disorders are the most common medical complication of pregnancy and childbirth.

▶ The so-called "childbearing years" are the most common time for women to become depressed. Or, as the U.S. National Institute of Mental Health Web site puts it, "Although conventional wisdom holds that depression is most closely associated with menopause, in fact, the childbearing years are marked by the highest rates of depression."

▶ A prior history of mood disorders is considered a risk factor for postpartum depression. But more than half of women with postpartum depression are experiencing a mood disorder for the first time.

▶ While postpartum disorders affect up to 25 per cent of new mothers, postpartum psychosis is relatively rare, affecting one to two mothers in a thousand. It just happens to attract more media attention.

WISE WORDS

"While parents-to-be receive considerable preparation for the physical aspects of birth, they are rarely prepared for the emotional challenges of parenthood, or given information about the stressors they may face. Thus, when disturbing feelings and events arise during the postpartum period, parents may be very surprised and unprepared. In the absence of information and support, they may conclude that their reactions are unusual, and reflective of their own inadequacies as parents. . . . The consequences are likely to be silence, an exacerbation of symptoms, and very frequently, relational conflicts."

— from "Not Just the Blues" by PASS-CAN, a charitable organization providing support to families across the country (www.passcan.ca).

SARAH HAMID
On Meds

Friday, November 15, 1996, after 10 p.m.:

I'm crying again in my room as I listen to Sarah McLachlan CDs and clutch an old teddy bear in the dark. The door is open, because I secretly want someone to find me, but the closest room is my grandmother's, and she's incredibly hard of hearing. My parents' room is on the far side of the house. It must be the hundredth consecutive day of crying, for no reason other than the doom-filled feeling that I am slowly falling off the edge of the world. At school, I cry into my sleeve at study carrels, in bathroom stalls, even in crowded lecture halls. I keep seeing words like "death" flashing in my mind's eye and resonating in my ears. I sleep fifteen hours a day, sneaking in lovely escapist naps when no one is looking, and I often think of the mercifulness of suicide. All this from a well-rounded, spiritual, and amiable straight-A student attending university on a $20,000 scholarship. If I, of all people, can't "think" away this thing in my head, who can?

My grandmother's numerology predictions always indicated that my eighteenth year would be very important. It turns out she was right. That November night, I couldn't stand the pain any more. I couldn't stand the hiding, all those times wearing sunglasses so no one would see me cry, weeping in showers and into towels and teddy bears. I hadn't told another living soul, just God in my prayers, about what I was going through. Praying several times a day gave me the strength not to kill myself, but it didn't help the symptoms. I needed human help desperately.

I started the journey to my mom's room a dozen times before I made it to her door and, still bawling, said the words: "Mommy, there's something wrong with me. I'm going crazy." I don't know how I mustered the courage, because I felt like such a failure. I felt all of six years old just then.

My mother was in her nightie and reading glasses, doing a crossword in bed. The second she heard my voice, she leaped into mom mode – just as she has always done. Running over to hold me, she asked what was wrong. I blubbered that I didn't know. She asked if I was feeling overwhelmed with school. I said, "I guess." I didn't want to tell her it was bigger than school, that school actually gave me distraction and purpose. How do you tell a mother that her otherwise healthy, vibrant eighteen-year-old daughter is overwhelmed by life?

Like her parents had done for her as a child in Bombay, my mom gave me some homeopathic pills to put under my tongue and relax me. Growing up, I had come to enjoy the candylike medicine and took it now as a salve. She also kicked my dad downstairs and made me sleep next to her. (I still don't know what she told him to justify his being bumped out of his own bed without alarming him too much.) At any rate, she knew just what I needed. My road to healing started that night.

On Monday, we went to see my family doctor. What a powerful advocate a concerned family member can be – Hell hath no fury like a worried mother! My mom related everything while I nodded and mumbled in agreement. The doctor finally started asking me questions about depression; he had completely neglected this possibility during all the recent visits I had paid to him for somatic complaints like headaches, sleepiness, and lack of appetite.

To rule out severe PMS, I was instructed to keep a mood diary for a month. During this time, I just kept getting worse. One day I cried for hours and hours, to the point that I ran out of tears and dry-sobbed while my abdominals spasmed with fatigue. If I had been injured and was unable to stop *bleeding*, the emergency room might have seemed an option, but this was a middle-class, suburban, immigrant household with no experience handling psychiatric emergencies. My parents and brother ran around the house in a panic trying to move my doctor's appointment up. While I was trying to listen to dance music in my bedroom to make the tears stop, I could hear my mom yelling with receptionists on the phone, almost threatening them to squeeze me in.

In the end, she dumped me in the car and raced to the doctor; I was crying the whole way there. I told the doctor that it was clear my moods were not connected to my period. After one last round of questions and blood tests, I was finally diagnosed with major unipolar depression.

Months later, I would learn that depression ran at least two generations back in my maternal line. (My mother suddenly realized during an episode of the TV show *Dr. Quinn, Medicine Woman* that "melancholia" was the same thing as "depression.") Apparently, her uncle had been institutionalized with the condition.

My father also had a short but deep bout of depression upon his arrival to Canada from Switzerland (and before that, a war-ravaged Afghanistan). Alone in Vancouver, unable to find a job, this otherwise articulate, educated, and physically impressive man was reduced to tears. He ultimately found solace in his faith and readings of the Koran. My father had always told me religion was like toothpaste: it comes in lots of different brand names and flavours but the function is the same, to cleanse the soul. My own spiritual faith gave me solace, too, solace that my suffering would end and ultimately serve some purpose. I couldn't or wouldn't believe God could do this to me for nothing.

But while God was working to help my soul, my doctor was working on my brain chemistry. I was immediately put on antidepressant Number 1, but it made me feel worse. Not only did it *not* help my illness, it added two caffeine-like side-effects: complete insomnia and the jitters. After a horrific week, I went off it and tried the pill behind Door Number 2. Almost immediately, I got better.

If some members of my extended family initially didn't believe how chemical this illness was for me, they were now starting to understand. "It must be hormones" was as chemical as their theories had ever been. I don't blame them, though. Growing up in India and Afghanistan doesn't expose you to a lot of dialogue on serotonin, dopamine, or neural synapses. I had grown up in Canada and knew something of the biological models of mental illness from pop culture and from my university psych courses.

Two weeks on the new drug, and the crying, my major symptom, disappeared. I went from having several episodes a day to none for two weeks. And then the crying came back. It seems I had responded beautifully to the drug but then plateaued. Like winning a silver at the Olympics, I felt so close and yet so frustratingly far. I begged my doctor to do something. He increased the dosage and added other drugs to my regimen, but I was still stuck at about 40 or 50 per cent better. And scared.

Should I settle for the $500 or see what's behind Door Number 3? Should I sacrifice the certainty of partial improvement on one drug for a new drug that offered a chance of greater recovery but also a risk of going back down to zero? In the end, I was not prepared to accept that 40 or 50 per cent was as good as I could expect. I took the risk. I'm a high achiever; I set high standards for myself in my academics, in my creative writing, in my various other activities (ballroom dancing, pottery), and in my health now too.

During this whole game of find-the-magical-chemical-cocktail, I was in second-year university doing a co-op term, and was employed as a work-at-home journalist. I also just happened to be falling in love for the first time. (It certainly doesn't wait for a convenient moment to find you.) Love rudely awakened me to the numbing effect that depression, and the drugs that are supposed to help it, can have on sexual thoughts and feelings. Luckily, I had landed myself a real sweetie, who saw *me* behind the grey haze, saw me at my absolute worst and loved me anyway.

Having tapped out the expertise of my GP, I began seeing a psychiatrist, after a long wait, to establish an antidepressant action plan. Over the next twenty months, I would go through another dozen drugs, dosages, and combinations. Each time my mom and I went to fill a new prescription, my heart brimmed with hope. And each time those expectations were dashed as my symptoms persisted and I suffered myriad side effects (dry mouth, nausea, jitters, sedation). Blood tests and ECGs became as regular as my doctor visits. My loving friends and family stood by, unable to do anything but hug me, as they watched me suffer through trial-and-error after trial-and-error. I cannot describe how physically and emotionally exhausting it was to ride the roller coaster of hope and side effects offered by each new array of pills. At the time, I was so depressed I underestimated the extent to which my family, best friend, and boyfriend suffered too. Now, in retrospect, I'm aware that their own mental health and spiritual strength were under constant strain.

Eventually I said "enough," and in October 1998 – more than two years after the symptoms had started and around the time a very close family member passed away – I finally asked to be put back on drug Number 2. (By this time, the manufacturer had come up with a new slow-release formulation of the drug.) A very high dose is what finally got me stable. Of course, there was no reason to expect better results the second time around; I just lucked out. I attribute that luck to divine intervention and a gift from the soul of my departed aunt, who had been like another mother to me.

Antidepressant medicine has saved my life in every sense of the word. I still have inexplicable crying jags, but only once every two months or so. Instead of lasting hours, they last ten or fifteen minutes. I used to be on 450 mg a day; now I'm at 225 and weaning down towards zero. I don't intend to stay medicated for life unless I have to, and my doctors believe that I won't need to. Part of me also wants to know whether the depression is in remission or just lurking around waiting for me to let my antidepressant guard down before it leaps out at me again. Sometimes in my excitement, I find I have weaned down a bit faster than I should have, resulting most recently in a major relapse. It's easy to forget that rehabilitation is not a straight line but a process of moving forwards, backwards, sideways.

To help me remember, I have undertaken short-term counselling, including cognitive-behavioural therapy, to give me the tools and space I need to cope with this relapse and the potential for future ones. I also needed to find some closure for the past six years. Living through a major mental illness and then making the painstaking journey back towards recovery is a traumatic, soul-shaking experience. It breaks you then rebuilds you, hopefully better than before. But there's no mistaking that first it broke me open to the very core.

So for now, medication keeps me stable. What keeps me *well* is attention to exercise, faith, sleep, nutrition, stress levels, and social supports. My social network has been great, especially my mom and my boyfriend, because they've physically been there during so many spells. They know exactly what to do: just listen and hold me. My dog is great at it, too. Touch from any loved one is so immediately therapeutic.

I'm twenty-four now and happier than I've ever been – even at 90-per-cent symptom-free. I don't dread the crying jags any more; in fact, I'm grateful for them, because they help remind me where I've been, how I've matured, and what the real priorities are in life. My illness has also been a key factor in securing and succeeding at my current occupation: communications co-ordinator at the Canadian Mental Health Association's British Columbia Division. Here, I find nourishment for the mind, hands, and soul, and work each day hoping that I can help just one person cope with their first episode of mental illness – or better yet, help just one person avoid it in the first place.

Sarah Hamid lives in Vancouver with her boyfriend of five years. She's written several autobiographical stories for the CMHA-BC *journal,* Visions.

THE STUDENT MIND/BODY

The Centre for Addiction and Mental Health in Toronto conducted surveys of several thousand elementary and high school students, university students, and adults in Ontario in 1998 and 1999.

▶ Of the three groups, university students are the most likely to indicate symptoms of depression, anxiety, or social dysfunction.

▶ Forty-nine per cent of university students reported feeling constantly under stress (versus 36 per cent of high school students and 21 per cent of adults).

▶ Female high school and university students are "significantly more likely to report poor mental health" than boys of the same age.

▶ The survey of adults found that the younger we are, the more likely we are to report high levels of psychological distress. Almost 18 per cent of the youngest group (ages eighteen to twenty-nine) did so, compared to less than 7 per cent of the oldest group (sixty-five and up).

THE DOCTOR WILL SEE YOU NOW . . .

▶ People are seeing their doctors for depression more and more frequently. The number of patient visits shot up 36 per cent between 1995 and 2000.

▶ Two-thirds of visits for depression were by women.

▶ Middle-aged people (aged forty to fifty-nine) were the most common visitors, followed by young adults (aged twenty to thirty).

▶ In the year 2000, Canadians filled 15.8 million prescriptions for antidepressant medications. That's up 60 per cent since 1996.

▶ In 2000, more than three million prescriptions for Paxil were filled in Canada, making it the country's most commonly prescribed antidepressant medication, and the eighth most commonly prescribed of all medications.

(All statistics from IMS Health's year-end statistics for 2000.)

MARGOT KIDDER
On Orthomolecular Medicine

Late April, 1996. You're gazing, blankly, at a television set on the ward of a psychiatric hospital in Los Angeles. You're exhausted, too, from the frenzy of the past few days. All that running and hiding, the CIA in hot pursuit. Who would ever have thought they'd send thirty-nine agents – and all for one woman!

You fooled them, though. Gave the CIA the slip and kept on running. Ran till you'd spent your last dime and blended in with L.A.'s homeless. Even slept in a cardboard box during your great escape. All of that, and more, you survived – only to be brought here. Back to the bin. *Shit*.

The TV set is droning away when suddenly an image commands your undivided (and horrified) attention. It's a picture of *you* – and the reporter is talking about how you've been taken to a psychiatric hospital for observation. You were found (looking a little "dishevelled," he says) in someone's backyard. He also says that some of your dental work was missing and suggests perhaps a good chunk of your mind is likewise unaccounted for.

Quick, flip the channel. *Damn*. More clips from one of the four *Superman* flicks you did with Christopher Reeve. Flip, flip, *damn*. It's on all the networks, the news channels, the entertainment shows. Everyone's talking about the former Lois Lane, and how she's now apparently right off her rocker.

Unfortunately, this part is no delusion. Nor is it a movie.

Fast-forward. It's April 2001, and Margie Kidder, looking radiantly healthy, is recalling that very painful moment. She is standing at a podium. And she's *smiling*.

"I was in the nuthouse, watching the news about my flip-out, thinking, 'This is a bad career move!'"

Kidder explodes with laughter – at her defiant use of the words "nuthouse" and "flip-out" and at her punchline. The audience, a group of several hundred who've come to hear her speak on the holistic brand of treatment she now lives by, roars its approval.

"But then, I didn't really have much of a career at that point," Kidder continues. "I'd pretty much ruined that with manic ups and downs and people going, 'Wow, *there's* a piece of work. She's kinda difficult, *even for movies*.'" More laughter at her self-deprecation. It's so *un*-movie-star-like.

This is vintage Kidder. The captivating honesty has audience members rolling with laughter one moment and reeling in shock the next. It's a bit like hitching a ride on a roller coaster.

Kidder likes that, seeing people moved by her story. She also likes seeing people learn from it, to hear that it's possible to be stable and happy and healthy using an alternative to mainstream psychiatric medication. At least it's worked for her. After a lifetime of ups and downs and "wig-outs," she's now been enjoying a long period of stability, peace, and joy.

"Doctors say, with cancer, if you go five years without a recurrence of the illness that you get to be called 'cured.' And this week, I had five years. And I'm calling myself 'cured.'"

Strong words. Encouraging words, prompting another burst of applause. Words that must be a tremendous relief to be able to say. Because Margie Kidder (that's her real name and the one she prefers) has struggled many times with the monster of bipolar affective disorder during her life, rocketing to outer space before plummeting straight to hell. She knows how hard it can be to claw out from that pit, its walls smooth and slippery, its bottom an infinite and lightless chasm.

To her tremendous credit, she's managed, every time, to make that difficult return trip. And now, finally, this once-frequent flyer is grounded, in the best sense of the word.

But her decision to reject mainstream psychiatric medication and pursue a therapy based on vitamins and minerals and balance throws some people for a loop. And that includes television personality Barbara Walters, who interviewed Kidder just two days before the conference.

"She greeted me with the most worried look on her face, going, 'Margot, are you all right? I've been so worried about you. I heard you're doing this alternative medicine.' And I went, 'I'm really well. I'm more well than I've been in my life, possibly since I was eleven.'"

Plagued with volatile moods since childhood, Kidder has tried just about every conventional psychiatric treatment in the book. (She's even toyed with some really oddball psychotherapies, one of which involved repeatedly smacking a pillow with a plastic bat while shouting 'I *hate* you Mommy! I *hate* you Mommy!' – a statement that wasn't even true.)

"I did 'em all. There wasn't a therapy I hadn't tried, and there wasn't a drug that I hadn't tried."

Unfortunately, none of it seemed to *work* for her. And so, from her twenties through her thirties and into her late forties, the woman who'd adopted the fake Hollywood name of Margot wrestled with sporadic mood swings that would wreak occasional havoc on her friendships, her marriages, her family life. It's little wonder that she entitled her (as-yet) unpublished autobiography *Calamities*. She's lived them.

To recount all of Kidder's ups and downs would be a bit like writing the biography of a slide whistle. Or, based on what she's revealed from *Calamities*, perhaps a postmodern melodrama: moments of rapturous joy and somersault love punctuated by periods of impossible and relentless pain. All of it, peppered with that trademark Kidder humour. Margie is a *very* funny lady.

She's also very gracious, agreeing to a total of three lengthy interviews. And of course, part of what *everyone* wants to know is a little more about what happened during that big, nasty, flip-out.

"It changed my life," she says simply. For the better.

This most public of manias occurred following a highly creative and productive period of memoir-writing. A computer virus began gnawing its way through her hard drive, devouring tens of thousands of words she'd poured her very soul into. In a panic, she took her computer (with more files vanishing every time she checked) to data recovery specialists. They told her she was out of luck.

The stress of losing all that work triggered a delusion that the virus had been deliberately planted because some very powerful people wanted the book destroyed. Before long, Kidder was convinced she was being followed – and that the lives of her sister and daughter were in jeopardy.

"I was literally all over L.A. for quite a few days," she recalls, "screaming at people, 'Get off my back! All these CIA agents for one middle-aged woman? How dare you, blah blah blah.' I was out there screaming, 'Just shoot me. Just get it over with. Blow me up, but don't prolong this.'"

Only those who've experienced a similar delusion could possibly relate to the feeling, but the *fear* was agonizing. Agents in unmarked cars lurked at every corner, relaying her whereabouts. Even bank machines had been rigged to explode if Kidder's card and PIN number were entered. Her only option was to try, with every ounce of strength and cunning and adrenalin she had, to abandon her identity and flee this omnipresent danger.

And so it came to be that a movie star known pretty much around the world wound up in a shantytown of poverty. Margot Kidder was, for several days, living with the homeless in a village of cardboard in the shadow of a grimy expressway.

"There were people from every walk of life there. At one point I said, 'I don't know how to act. I'm not from this part of town.' And this fellow said to me, '*None* of us are from this part of town.' So it was very humbling."

Humbling, too, because many strangers – out of the goodness of their hearts – simply gave. A man named Charlie shared his cardboard box because Margie had nowhere else to sleep; someone else gave her sandwiches they'd collected from a convenience store (which couldn't sell them once their "best before" date had expired). A woman who saw Kidder wearing a filthy garbage bag (a disguise to fool the agents), pulled over her car and gave her a coffee and some money. She drove away, only to return a short time later with clean clothes. All this, despite the fact Kidder looked and sounded like a madwoman.

"She never said anything negative: she just gave. And every one of those things that happened allowed me to stay in the human loop, so that I wasn't completely isolated and out there," she says.

When eventually taken to hospital, Kidder was desperate to try a different path to wellness. She challenged her involuntary status and appeared before a judge. She was still higher than a kite, but a close friend gave the following advice: 'You're an actress. *Act.*'

"And so I did one of the best acting jobs of my career, in that I pretended I was sane. And the judge said, 'You're free to go.'"

With the help of her brother, arrangements were made for her to spend time recovering on Vancouver Island with a woman who specializes in acupuncture and other holistic treatments. A large part of the approach was to allow Kidder to come to her own terms with what had taken place. In those early, post-hospital days, the actor was consumed with trying to determine whether the delusion that had seemed so real actually was. The acupuncturist offered an interesting opinion.

"She said to me, 'Well, you might never know. Perhaps it was real; perhaps it wasn't, on an objective, existential level. But your body went through it and your mind went through it and your emotions went through it, therefore *you* went through it. Therefore, let us heal you from the trauma of what you experienced, because it was real to you.'"

That simple truth, Kidder says, prompted a realization that her single most important task was to recover from the trauma of the ordeal. To allow her body, mind and soul to calm themselves after having endured some three weeks in a constant fight-or-flight mode. And so, with the help of acupuncture and peaceful surroundings, Kidder allowed herself to sleep. Or to weep, grieving over what she'd been through. Or simply to reflect.

She returned home to Montana to find that tabloid photographers were on the hunt for the first photo of Lois Lane from la-la-land. Zoom lenses were everywhere.

"They were going to get a picture of me looking demented if it killed them. It was a very difficult way to get well, with reporters chasing you around and snapping pictures inside the window of my house."

On the other hand, Kidder was tremendously touched by the mail that arrived every day. Loving, supportive letters from around the world that told her she was not alone.

"Every letter started basically the same way," she says. " 'I've never told anyone this – this is a secret my family has kept forever – but . . .'

"And it began to be clear to me that half of the horror of it was keeping the secret, and that half the horror of it was that none of us in society would admit that this was a very common thing, that almost every family has been through some sort of episode of somebody in the family falling apart."

The letters reinforced Kidder's determination not only to get well, but to *stay* well. And so began the homework. In short order, the actor gathered a small library of books on bipolar affective disorder, including dense academic works by neurologists. She picked up a medical dictionary and a chemistry dictionary and a biology dictionary. And then, for pretty much an entire year, she read. And the more she read, the more she believed there were other, more natural ways of keeping things on an even keel. Including the relationship between diet and mood.

"I used to live on hot dogs and Diet Coke. Never once did a shrink ever say to me, 'What do you eat?' And none of them ever mentioned that sleeping might be a good idea," she says with disbelief.

It wasn't long before Kidder had become a convert to a still-controversial branch of therapy known as orthomolecular medicine. At its essence, the treatment uses megadoses of vitamins and minerals, plus solid nutrition, to restore and maintain a state of balance: toxins out, good stuff in. Mainstream psychiatry doesn't pay a whole lot of attention to the field, and some argue that high doses of certain vitamins can be damaging.

Proponents, however, say the risk is small compared with the potential side effects of many major psychiatric medications. They also believe that the reason this movement has never cracked the mainstream is because there's little in it for the drug companies. You can't patent vitamins.

People like Kidder say they've found stability with a combination of orthomolecular medicine and a healthy lifestyle; others use it as an adjunct to their regular treatment. And though the actor uses a cascade of four-letter words in describing her own experience with psychiatric drugs, she insists she knows they serve an important role.

"I'm not anti-drug. I'm anti the *abuse* of these drugs. Yes, they're useful a lot of the time. But they shouldn't be useful to the point where they become all the treatment there is for all mental illnesses with nothing else. And that's really the big problem."

A problem, she says, because human beings are unique: so incredibly complex that the labels and treatment that fit one person aren't necessarily right for someone else with similar symptoms. Yet Kidder insists that psychiatry tends to use what she calls the "throw the drug at the label" approach.

"You could have five people who've been diagnosed with manic depression and they could have five different problems. So the conventional psychiatric approach is, excuse my language, crazy."

Every chance she gets, Kidder stresses that she's not telling people to throw out their pills. Rather, she's asking them to consider the possibility that alternatives can work. To do their own research. To open their minds and – now that she knows what it's like to be homeless – their hearts.

"I do know," she says, "that amongst the homeless and the downtrodden and those poor people, there are some brilliant, wonderful, incredible people. And we as a society have chosen to ignore that. We've chosen to separate; we make this big wall between well and okay – and mentally ill."

That wall, she says, should not exist.

"There's none of us with an absolutely clean, innocent soul, who doesn't have some dark shadow parts in our psyches. We all have those.

"Next time you pass someone who's homeless and crazy, give them two bucks. Don't walk on the other side of the street. They're not a bad person. They deserve respect. The lady on the street corner yelling at the phantoms deserves our respect. Because she's made it through a lot of shit and she's still standing."

Kidder, who has a long history of social activism (that's how she wound up dating former prime minister Pierre Trudeau), now divides her time between acting and advocating. She speaks frequently at major conferences throughout North America and takes occasional roles on television and in movies.

During one of her recent gigs, a guest spot on *Law and Order*, she was filming in New York. Her wallet was stolen and she contacted the police. They suggested, logically, she search the garbage bins near where she thought the theft had occurred.

"And I was walking along Madison Avenue, going through the garbage, and I went, 'No, Kidder. Not with your image. This is *not a* good thing.'" She lets out another burst of laughter as she imagines the tabloid headlines.

Computer technicians managed to recover most of the data from Calamities, *and Kidder now uses virus protection software. She's also thinking about writing another book; this one, a user-friendly manual on orthomolecular medicine. (Plus, of course, a little something on that wig-out.)*

BIPOLAR DISORDER

▶ The best estimate reached by the Surgeon General's 1999 report on mental health in the United States is that 1.7 per cent of the population has bipolar disorder in any given year.

▶ It can clearly take time for correct diagnosis of a mood disorder. According to the Toronto-based Centre for Addiction and Mental Health, 29 per cent of patients with mood disorders reported that it took more than ten years to receive a correct diagnosis. Sixty per cent said they'd received an incorrect diagnosis in the past.

▶ Research shows that 50 to 60 per cent of people with bipolar disorder also have a substance abuse or dependence problem.

▶ Genetic research still hasn't found any gene or genes responsible for bipolar disorder. But most researchers believe there is a genetic component because of findings from family studies. A Health Canada report notes: "The prevalence rate of bipolar disorder among first-degree relatives of patients with bipolar disorder is estimated to be 7.5%, five to ten times higher than in the general population" (*A Critical Review of the Literature on Children at Risk for Major Affective Disorders*, 1995).

▶ Unlike unipolar depression, most of whose sufferers are female, bipolar disorder is equally common in women and men.

LESLIE CÔTÉ
On Film-making

The first time we meet Leslie Côté, her hair is pure blond and almost to her waist. Two weeks later, it's a rich auburn-red skimming her shoulders. The dramatic change is a reflection of her life, which is everywhere in transition. Côté is buying a new house, packing up the old one, and travelling the country directing episodes for a new thirteen-part television series.

Throughout, she is casually chic, as only a thirty-something native Montrealer can be. Dressed in black leather pants and heeled boots, with matching hat, scarf, and gloves, she carries all the essential accoutrements of a woman on the go: Palm Pilot, cellphone, Day-Timer. Put it all together and she cuts a striking figure, whatever the colour of her hair.

A newspaper article about the documentary she has co-directed and co-produced has brought her to our attention. In the accompanying photo, Côté looks tall and healthy and confident. Yet there she is, in print, revealing she'd lived for ten years with an eating disorder.

After a flurry of phone calls and e-mails, she agrees to speak with us about her film and her life.

"I wanted to make the film," she begins, "to prove that eating disorders were not simply about the pressures from magazines to look thin. That somehow it was rooted in some kind of trauma." She and co-director/producer Felicia Francescut put an ad in a Toronto newspaper, interviewed about three dozen women who responded to it, then picked three to follow around for several months. The filmmakers became subjects, too, revealing their own past disorders on-camera. The key word there is *past*: Côté was convinced she'd long since learned everything there was to know about her own illness and recovery.

"I don't think I thought I would learn anything I hadn't already talked about in my own therapy. My motives were altruistic." She's smiling, as she says this, at her own conceit. Her initial goal had been to help viewers see the "naked truth" about anorexia, bulimia, and overeating. But life, as they say, is what happens when you're making other plans. And the process of piecing together her documentary wound up helping the filmmaker as much as anyone.

"Making this film helped me to heal in a way that I never expected," she says now. "It opened a different avenue for looking at some of the issues in my own life."

SCENE: *A large woman named Elka emerges from a clothing-store dressing room in a long, clingy dress that reveals her abundant round-ness. Bumps and lumps and folds of flesh – what she calls her "bowling balls" – are exposed for all to see. "This is my worst night-mare," she says. "This is it. This is the dress that makes me leave stores after going shopping and go directly to my bed with a pastrami sand-wich and a pack of cigarettes that I can smoke in about an hour."*

SCENE: *A small, short-haired woman named Susan steps onto a doctor's scale, telling the film-makers not to show the number she weights in at. She is so frail – so seemingly devoid of muscle, fat, or fluid – that viewers surely wonder if her weight will register at all. She looks tense, almost trapped, and promptly explains why. "I prefer to be closer to eighty," she says. (That's pounds.) "I'm embarrassed at how heavy I am."*

SCENE: *A fit-looking young woman named Mary Kay lists off her daily teaching schedule: aquafitness, boxing circuit, step-and-sculpt classes. She is cute and blonde. She's also been bulimic for fifteen years, with a total of two years spent in hospital. "One day I might feel like binging and puking, and it might be because me and the girl at work got into a bit of a tiff," she says plainly. "One day, I might feel like it because I don't feel good enough."*

Through Thick and Thin: The Naked Truth about Eating Disorders does precisely what this book attempts to do: it pulls at the barriers that conspire to separate people with disorders from the rest of the world. After all, who hasn't thought, during those inevitable dark moments in life, "I don't feel good enough," as Mary Kay says? Eating disorders are one part of that vast spectrum of methods – some healthy, others not – we use to deal with those feelings. "Some people work through it, developing symptoms that are more obvious," Côté says. "Others work through it and develop symptoms that we don't even as a society recognize as symptoms."

She and Francescut wanted to find women willing to explore these issues. Côté was particularly interested in how childhood experiences might be connected to adult disorder. She'd done ten years of psychotherapy exploring those connections in her own life, and had even taken training to become a therapist herself. Now, as part of the film, she'd have to delve back into her past with the same kind of honest self-reflection Elka, Susan, and Mary Kay were offering.

SCENE: *Leslie stands naked before a blank white wall, writing extracts on it from her journal. "For ten years of my life I starved myself to the point of dizziness, I ate until I felt sick, and I took laxatives to rid myself of the sins of a binge," she writes.*

Leslie's symptoms progressed in a familiar pattern: dieting and exercise in high school leading to diet pills, caffeine pills, uppers. The worst of it started when, at sixteen, she moved away to boarding school. By university, she'd added laxatives to the mix, the purging part of the binge-and-purge cycle that is bulimia. "You binge because you're having a feeling, and you can't stand the feeling. Then after the binge, you feel guilty, so you purge to rid yourself of the sins of the binge," she explains. "Eating disorders are about needing to control the body, because you feel out of control in other places in your life."

Côté's early life was one of seeming privilege. Raised in the wealthy Montreal neighbourhood of Westmount, she grew up with expensive vacations, beautiful clothes, regular trips to New York. Her mother was English-speaking, her father French Canadian. Leslie switched between French and English schools, feeling she never quite fitted in. "I really struggled to just find a place where I could be accepted." Somewhere along the way, being accepted became equated with being pretty, and especially being thin. Like many teenagers, she was struggling to find an identity separate from her mother's. Bulimia became the secret she guarded. "I wanted to be different than my mother . . . but I didn't know who to be. So I feel that in some senses I clung to this bulimia as an identity."

And she clung to it for many years. Along with the binging and purging and self-starvation, there were suicidal thoughts as well as depression. In the film, she depicts this inner torment with graphic images of herself, naked, bound by heavy cloth, or chained to a refrigerator, or leaning over a toilet bowl with a noose around her neck. "I had a love-hate relationship with food," she says to the camera. "A relationship of extremes. A direct reflection of how I felt about myself."

When filming began, Côté still had not shared the painful details of her illness with her mother. And her silence on this one subject continued to separate them.

SCENE: *An old black-and-white photograph shows Leslie as a teenager, looking moody in dark sunglasses. "My mother and I talk from time to time," her adult voice narrates. "We're not all that close, though."*

Each of the film's subjects has a troubled relationship with her mother. Susan's is the most overt. "My mother tried to beat the good into us," she tells the film-makers. From the ages of ten to twelve, Susan reveals, she was sexually abused by someone outside her family, and was also physically abused by her mother. "I was terrified, absolutely terrified, that I was going to have a baby," she says. "And terrified not that I was going to have a baby, [but] that my mother would kill me."

Elka, from earliest childhood, loved to sing. On camera, she describes how her mother's dream was to see her sing at the Metropolitan Opera. When young Elka's voice deepened from soprano to mezzo-soprano, her mother was horrified. "Mezzos aren't Butterfly . . . or Violetta!" Elka remembers her saying. Elka's world "imploded, and I felt sucked down a drain. I stopped singing. . . . So I ate. . . . What else do you do? There were very few things in my life that made me feel really free."

In one of the film's most revealing scenes, Mary Kay sits with her mother in the family living room. She is enraged, but unable to articulate the source of that rage. "You treated me with anger," she spits out. Then she starts to cry. "It's too intellectual with you, Mom. You never talk about it." Her mother silently absorbs the shock waves. Then she reaches for her daughter's hand. "*I just don't understand*," Mary Kay whispers. Their eyes do not meet.

In that same living room, from the other side of the camera, Leslie Côté took in the anger, the obvious rift between mother and daughter. What she saw that day was herself reflected. It was a pivotal moment in her life. "What I became aware of was that I had my own anger around my mother that I had not quite worked through, and that, like Mary Kay, I was still blaming my mother for my eating disorder."

She saw, too, that anger and blame were only part of the picture. Home video of Mary Kay as a girl, splashing in the family swimming pool with her mother, hinted at a once-intimate, even playful, relationship. "You see a certain camaraderie, a certain spirit, a connection between them." And this, too, for Côté, was cause for self-reflection.

Before shooting began, Côté had made a promise to her mother: Whichever pieces of her story she chose to reveal on-camera, she would be "coming from a good place." She'd been grappling with that promise ever since. "It took me a long time to figure out what I was saying [with the words] 'I'm coming from a good place.' It took me a very long time to understand that that meant I can't blame her for this, that I had to look at my own responsibility. . . . I never really understood that laying blame was not taking responsibility. I don't think that ever really sunk in until I was making this film. *I* made that choice to starve myself and binge."

As filming progressed, a dialogue began away from the cameras. For the first time, Leslie Côté and her mother began to talk openly about the symptoms she'd lived with – and the feelings that went with them – throughout her teens and early twenties. At thirty-five, she was finally sharing her secret.

SCENE: *"When my mother and I spoke recently about the bulimia, she was curious about what had happened," Leslie writes on the wall. "She asked questions and then quietly listened. I was surprised. I feared judgment, but instead she showed compassion for the shame that I had carried with me for years."*

"I'm glad I made the film," Côté says now. "I might have learned this lesson in a different way, at a different point in time. [But] everything has a reason for presenting itself when it presents itself."

So much of Leslie Côté's early life was consumed with the need to escape her own emotions. When, with the help of therapy, she finally gave up purging, her binging only intensified; waking from a nightmare, she'd steal downstairs and raid the fridge. In desperation, she once resorted to placing a padlock on the fridge door, asking her roommate to hide the key each night. Then, coming downstairs and being confronted by the lock, she'd throw a coat over her nightgown and drive to an all-night food store.

Through therapy – from psychotherapy to art therapy, group therapy, meditation, and bioenergetic work – she's learned to cope with emotions in healthier ways. "Getting over it for me is really just about learning to feel the feelings and say, 'Okay, but that doesn't have to control me. It doesn't control my behaviour.'"

Filming her own scenes naked – as did her co-producer – was her personal statement that she had finally gained control. "Taking away that outer layer meant that we were exposed not just emotionally but also physically," she says. "It's ironic: people with eating disorders aren't connected to their bodies. They don't listen to their cues. And here we were, on the other hand, saying we *are* connected to our bodies and we're going to feel the emotions that we have while we're doing it. It was a very powerful experience."

For Côté, the final step in her own recovery came during editing, often one of the most stressful stages of filmmaking. "Felicia asked me, 'Do you think you'll ever be entirely rid of the eating disorder?'

And I said, 'When I quit smoking.' . . . That was the one thing I was doing that was a form of addiction. It's an appetite suppressant. And it's a crutch, an emotional crutch."

During a meditation workshop, she found herself reaching into her pockets and handing over her cigarettes. She hasn't smoked since.

The last time Leslie Côté called us, she was on her way to a funeral; her father had died unexpectedly. She was upset, obviously. But her voice sounded strong. She knew what she needed to do, how to see herself through.

"Through Thick and Thin" aired on CBC *Newsworld's* The Passionate Eye. *It has won many awards and been shown at several film festivals, including the prestigious Banff Film Festival.*

On the eve of her father's death, Côté's film was nominated for a Gemini Award for best writing in a documentary program or series.

EATING DISORDERS

▶ Eating disorders affect an estimated seventy million people worldwide.

▶ The U.S. National Association of Anorexia Nervosa and Associated Disorders (ANAD) estimates that in the United States roughly seven million women and one million men have an eating disorder.

▶ An ANAD study of high school seniors concluded that 11 per cent have anorexia or bulimia.

▶ Anorexia nervosa kills twelve times more adolescent girls than all other causes combined (National Eating Disorder Information Centre — NEDIC).

▶ A U.S. study found that young girls are more afraid of becoming fat than of cancer, nuclear war, or losing their parents.

▶ Up to 80 per cent of Canadian teenaged girls feel "fat" even though they are not overweight, according to the NEDIC.

▶ Approximately 15 per cent of college women suffer from bulimia (NEDIC).

▶ A recent Ontario survey of more than 1,700 girls aged twelve to eighteen found that 27 per cent have disordered eating attitudes and behaviours that can lead to anorexia or bulimia. Rates increased with age.

IAN CHOVIL
On Work and Money

The story of Ian Chovil is, on a number of levels, a paradox.

Here's a guy who thought he was the world's most powerful man. In reality, he was homeless and destitute. Here's a cautionary tale that illustrates just about everything that can go wrong – and everything that can go right. Here's a story that travels through the lows of psychosis, addiction, and poverty before ending with recovery.

For Ian, the first half of that story is a nightmare the forty-eight-year-old would not wish on anyone: a decade of untreated psychosis.

"My acne was just disappearing," he says, "when I started getting the first symptoms. An insidious, gradual onset of symptoms."

The early symptoms were, relatively speaking, small potatoes. Some social withdrawal, a slight dip in ambition. Subtle enough they did not prevent Chovil from earning a double B.Sc. (honours) in biology and anthropology, or from attending graduate school in Halifax. That, however, is where delusions began to intrude. Strange beliefs that somehow didn't seem so strange to Ian.

Ian shared some of his odd thoughts (such as a conviction he was infected with a rare form of syphilis) with workers at a local health clinic. More powerful delusions (like the telepathic communication he was receiving from Jim Jones, the man responsible for a mass suicide in Guyana) he kept to himself.

"I would never admit to anyone what I was experiencing," he says.

And that may be why no one mentioned a diagnosis of schizophrenia, even though a psychiatrist he was referred to in Halifax prescribed an antipsychotic. Chovil took the medication briefly, hated its side effects, and stopped. Before long, school also stopped for Ian. He drifted westward to British Columbia, plunging free-fall into psychosis.

The many delusions that plagued Ian were highly intricate and, to him, exceedingly real. When homeless in Calgary in 1980, he believed he had caused the explosion of Mt. St. Helens with his mental powers. (The purpose of bringing about this cataclysm was to take pressure off the tectonic plates – thus preventing San Francisco from falling into the ocean.) He believed a Second World War veteran had followed him to the small B.C. town of Crofton. Unfortunately, the veteran had friends, and no matter where Ian went they'd find him. It made no difference that he spent nearly eight months bouncing through Alberta, staying in hostels, sleeping in ditches: the delusions followed.

In Victoria, he studied Buddhism under a Tibetan lama. The Tibetan actually *was* real, but his teachings meshed with, and enhanced, Ian's delusions. "He was a refugee from Tibet," Chovil remembers, "and he said, 'You special.' His English wasn't very good."

But special is certainly how Ian Chovil felt. So special that when the veteran told him to buy a gun, he purchased an army-surplus rifle. So special that, on many occasions, he sat in the basement with the barrel of the gun in his mouth.

"I would do that quite a lot, actually," he says.

After four years of living in abject poverty (and near-absolute psychosis), Chovil left Victoria in 1985, moved to Toronto, and landed a mind-numbing job changing lightbulbs in a large department store. His delusions, as before, tagged along. One of them spurred him to fly to Britain to meet the Maharishi Mahesh Yogi, where Ian was convinced he'd be welcomed as part of a sacred inner circle. The yogi, unfortunately, wasn't home.

"I flew back the next day," he says, managing a weak smile. "I spent $2,000 for a weekend in England."

Seeking to escape his delusions, his isolation, and the monotony of lightbulb-changing, Ian began to drink. What started with a single bottle of champagne to celebrate New Year's would, over time, escalate to a destructive routine. "I would get off work, drink a dozen beers, pass out, wake up in the morning, and go to work," he says. "My behaviour became more and more bizarre in that period. The combination of schizophrenia and substance abuse didn't mix very well." (Roughly half of all people with schizophrenia develop a substance abuse problem in their lifetime.)

As his psychosis deepened, a plethora of alien signs began revealing themselves: embedded in licence-plate numbers, in songs, even in the wall. Chovil was convinced he was on a mission to *become* an alien and survive the extinction of humanity. All the evidence was there – he had been chosen.

"I was the most important man in human history, because I was going to propagate the human species," he says. "My actual situation by then contrasted sharply. I was living in an illegal downtown rooming house, with only cockroaches for friends, working at this dumb job changing light bulbs five days a week, seven-and-a-half hours a day."

One night in 1987, angry at the aliens, he smashed several windows at his rooming house. The police took him to jail. "Prison was actually nicer than almost all the emergency shelters I have stayed at. We care more about our criminals than we do our homeless," he says dryly. A judge sentenced him to three years' probation, with the condition that he see a psychiatrist. Yet once again, due to the depths of his delusions, Chovil chose not to reveal to physicians the privileged mission he was on.

His alcohol abuse progressed, and he was dismissed from his job. He went from unemployment insurance to welfare, eventually brewing his own beer in plastic pails to save money. He also descended further into poverty, walking (because he couldn't afford the bus) to a variety of soup kitchens for free meals. He ate at one particular mission every day for an entire year.

One night in 1990, when other tenants at his rooming house began mainlining heroin in the living room, Ian could ignore his reality no longer. "I was blacking out a lot, waking up in strange places and getting these command hallucinations to buy beer with the rent money. I was a couple of months behind in the rent, and I knew I was going to become homeless soon." He accepted a psychiatrist's recommendation that he go to the Homewood Health Centre in Guelph for treatment of alcoholism.

As sobriety kicked in, many of the delusions, which had been exacerbated by the alcohol abuse, got kicked out. Chovil started to realize he had no concrete proof of aliens. Other unusual thoughts faded to nothing when he began a regular dose of antipsychotics.

One might reasonably think Chovil accepted the medication as a respite from his illness, from the delusions that had stolen so much. In fact, he took the drugs hoping they might bring an end to his *poverty*.

"It was the main reason I went on medication. It had nothing to do with anything else. Grinding poverty for me was always running out of money to do my laundry. And I would always feel really bitter when I got down to counting my quarters and dimes to see if I had enough money to do my laundry. I don't know exactly why, but it was the hardest part of my experience."

Ian did not, at this stage, actually accept that he had schizophrenia, but he was acutely aware of the abject poverty in which he'd been living. He says it would take three years "to really understand that I had schizophrenia and what that meant."

Recovering from long-term psychosis is hard enough. Yet already, Chovil was longing for something more meaningful than just mental stability, longing for a world beyond the confines of his small basement apartment in Guelph.

"I was very anxious," he says, "having nothing to do, and no one to do it with. I was really anxious, lonely, miserable, lethargic, and poor. Being stabilized on medication is not an indication of quality of life, really."

That anxiety led to a depression Chovil found was not alleviated by meds. On Sundays, he used to make a weekly trip to the corner store to buy a chocolate bar. The true motivation was a craving for something far more nourishing – human contact. Even, he says, if that contact consisted solely of: "That'll be $1.19 please. Thank you very much."

"I think that's the worst thing," he reflects. "The actual social isolation that comes with schizophrenia. It's just a phenomenal thing to be alone. With no job, no school, no friends, no lovers."

Rebuilding was not an overnight process. He found that a day treatment program, which often consisted of playing cards or Scrabble, wasn't much better than staying in the basement. The main benefit was connecting with some new friends, mostly other men with schizophrenia. Although he valued the companionship, Chovil and his new pals were all acutely aware of their situations. Schizophrenia had robbed precious years during a period when most people build careers, families, get on with their lives. The men in this group had little money and, or so they felt, even less appeal.

"So we'd see a group of women, and we'd think, Well, what are we going to say? 'Hi, I have schizophrenia and I'm on disability.' I mean, there was no way you could approach or talk to anybody. You feel like a real loser, no one would ever want to talk to you."

The same self-doubts would haunt them when it came to applying for employment.

"You have this long period where you haven't worked, and some people had schizophrenia before they'd even finished high school. You had no resumé, you had no employment skills – it was pretty horrible."

Chovil also found it pretty horrible trying to scrape by on disability benefits. Like many folks with mental disorders, Chovil is a smoker. Once he'd paid his rent, stocked up on groceries, and bought his cigarettes, there was barely anything left. Nor was there an abundance of opportunities.

And so Chovil decided, out of necessity, to create his own. With the help of a case manager, he started out delivering flyers to supplement his monthly benefits. It was actually pretty heavy work, carrying around a couple of thousand pieces of advertising that no one wanted. Burdensome, too, in other ways.

"I had to swallow my pride a lot. I'd graduated from university, I was in graduate school, and I'd always expected a professional career of one sort of another. And here I was, with one of the lowest jobs possible."

Nonetheless, Chovil was not deterred. He went from delivering flyers to delivering the local newspaper; he also began tinkering with computers and volunteering at the local cable station. Before long, he pitched a proposal for a television series on the mental health system. Soon, he was hosting his own monthly cable show.

"And it meant instant fame and notoriety in the mental health system," he recalls. People began asking Chovil to join various boards and committees. "It just kinda snowballed after the television thing."

Chovil initiated a series of well-received high school lectures, where he told students about his experience with schizophrenia. He then successfully lobbied the Homewood to give him a part-time position in community education that paid a modest honorarium. He has since been hired on as a permanent, half-time staff member, giving a considerable boost to his income. Wealth, however, is both a relative and subjective term. "Being paid for something is a real statement of what your value is."

After waiting seven years, Chovil finally got a subsidized apartment. He says the better home (with rent geared to income) and the extra cash have meant an incredible boost to his quality of life. He's been able to afford a used car, and has started to indulge in a newly acquired passion for top-notch audio equipment. He can also afford to buy better groceries than in the past.

Before the staff job, he says, "I had the same meal every night. It would be half a pound of ground beef, a third of a cup of rice, frozen mixed vegetables, a little margarine on the rice, a little ketchup on the lean ground beef, and that's it. And I had that every night for about five years."

Chovil is also pleased to now be able to travel freely to the United States, a freedom many people with serious mental illness have been denied in the past. Under existing rules, people with schizophrenia or manic depression, especially if they're unemployed, can be refused entry. Being able to say where he works means the question "And why *don't* you have a job?" never comes up.

But while these kinds of tangible gains – the car, the groceries, the stereo – have improved Ian's quality of life, he emphasizes that they are, ultimately, just things. And the most important thing to Chovil is worth far more than his paycheque.

"In more philosophical terms, working gives me more satisfaction in being human. I'm actually fairly happy being a human being these days."

Ian remains dedicated to public education, and his Web site, www.chovil.com, receives hundreds of curious visitors every day. He's been honoured with several prestigious awards in the mental health arena, plus a recent Mayor's Award of Excellence in Guelph. He continues to give roughly fifty presentations on his experience with schizophrenia every year in the hope others will learn, both from his misfortune and his recovery. He's become something of an ambassador for the illness, showing that with the right attitude – and the latest generation of medications – much can be accomplished.

After a decade in psychosis, it has not been an easy road back. But Chovil, to his credit, has paved it himself.

"Opportunities in the community are something a lot of people with mental illness don't have," he says. "If you'd asked me six or seven years ago, I would have said there was no point in continuing to live. And things have worked out pretty well.

"Like a friend of mine says, the plane is supposed to land in Florida but it winds up in Siberia. You can either be angry or you can accept where you've landed. These days, Siberia is quite pleasant."

In spring of 2002, Ian Chovil boarded a jet to Houston, where he was being interviewed on a major talk show. U.S. customs was a breeze.

ON (AND OFF) THE JOB

▶ According to a study by the U.S. National Alliance for the Mentally Ill, 85 per cent of people with serious mental disorders are unemployed.

▶ Research in Indiana indicates that people with severe mental illness show a reduction in symptoms and an increase in self-esteem when they are given competitive, challenging work. Those in a sheltered workshop (a non-competitive environment, usually involving low pay and unskilled labour) showed no such improvement.

▶ In Ontario, a freedom-of-information request revealed that more than 100,000 people are collecting from the province's disability support program because of mental illness or psychiatric disorder. That's nearly *two-thirds* of everyone receiving support under the plan.

▶ One Canadian study showed that when people with serious mental illness either work or are involved in meaningful activity, their self-reported rates of hospitalization plummeted from forty-eight days per year to just over four days per year. That represents a minimum saving in hospital expenses, per person, of $22,000 annually.

JOAN HAY
On Overcoming Stigma

On one wall of her home office, Joan Hay has hung, just below her college diploma and her two university degrees, the piece of paper that committed her to a psychiatric ward in 1996.

"I framed it in a certificate frame," she says with a wry smile. "It's matted. And it's signed. . . . It almost, to me, looks like a piece of art."

It's also a statement, a reminder that what we've overcome is every bit as important as what we have accomplished. Now a high school teacher working with students who have learning disabilities, Hay has told few of her colleagues or friends about her "psychiatric history." She worries, like pretty much everyone who's been where Joan has been, about being judged. And yet, there's the hospital certificate on display for anyone to see. Interesting thing is, nobody does. "People come in. They look. They look at that one, and they look at the others," Hay says. "And *they don't see it*." It's as if no one can believe that a woman possessing a diploma in recreation and degrees in English literature and education – to say nothing of a tall and athletic presence – could ever have been considered mentally ill.

And yet, she was – considered ill enough, in fact, to be locked up for two weeks. She's still struggling with the ever-present issue of who deserves, or needs, or can be trusted to know such things. "It's such a huge part of my life. And only a few people know," says Hay, thirty-six. "Part of me wants people to know, to try to break the stigma. But the other part is very much from my father, you know: Don't say anything, don't tell anybody."

Telling her story here, then, is a major decision – bigger even than deciding to display that certificate on the wall. Choosing to fight stigma is, for Hay and many others, an important step in her own recovery.

Hay became "officially ill," as she puts it, in 1994 while in the final year of her B.A. She'd been struggling for months, barely able to get herself to class and home again. As she was working on her very last essay, the bottom fell out. Scarcely able to sleep or eat, she spent several days staring endlessly at a blank computer screen and smoking cigarettes. In the end, she felt so wretched that she summoned the courage to call the number on a card she'd been carrying around for two months. It bore the name of a psychotherapist. "Something had to be done," Hay says. "But little did I know what I was in for."

The therapist – a kind woman who listened, empathized, and repeatedly asked "why" – advised Joan that she'd likely feel worse before she could feel better. And over the next year and a half, that's exactly what happened. "You start to investigate all these buried feelings, and things that I didn't know were buried," Hay says. "It came to the point where the pain was so intense I couldn't bear it."

Hay had been socially ill at ease since childhood, but now she completely withdrew. "I started getting terrible nightmares, not being able to sleep, not really caring about my appearance, not returning calls. *Really* not wanting to talk to anyone. I couldn't. I didn't want people to know how I was. I was embarrassed."

At night, she'd play suitably gloomy music – Joni Mitchell was a favourite – and tuck into a bottle of wine, for comfort. It was the only way she could feel okay. "And then one night . . . I had the music on and I was doing my nails, and I just kind of thought, Oh. *Oh!* And I started cutting myself. Not a clue what I was doing." What she was doing, in fact, was a well-recognized symptom of distress that psychiatrists now call self-injury (and until recently called self-harm). For Joan, it filled a need. "I needed to see the pain," she explains. "It was a total release."

Joan called a friend, who took her to the local hospital, where she waited several hours for a brief and unhelpful visit with an emergency-room doctor. It was, she says, "the worst time of my life." Her therapist would later say it was also the start of Joan's healing, a turning point of sorts.

None of this was known to the audience watching Joan perform at a local theatre the following night. Hay had joined a local comedy troupe specializing in Star Trek spoofs. (She'd been involved in amateur theatre for years, and had even considered moving to New York to try her hand as a professional; with her frank, self-deprecating humour, she might well have succeeded.) Despite what she'd recently endured, she did not want to let down her troupe members. "I had, of course, marks all along my arm," she recalls. "I don't know how I did it. I really don't. . . . I thought, this is so bizarre; I'm up here [on stage] and *no one* knows."

Over the next year and a half, Hay started seeing a psychiatrist as well as her psychotherapist, and was in and out of the hospital psych ward – how many times, she cannot even say. "Let's just say, they got to know me very well." Diagnosed with depression and anxiety, doctors prescribed ever-increasing dosages of anti-anxiety drugs, anti-depressants, and mood stabilizers before shipping her off home, where she would soon resume her evening ritual of lighting candles, drinking wine, and cutting. "It got to the point that I was becoming institutionalized. I didn't know or trust myself on the outside," she says. While on the inside, she felt completely removed from the world beyond the hospital. She remembers gazing out the window of the patient lounge, watching the seemingly happy people in the park below, and wondering how they could function out there.

Hay also spent longer stretches inside a psychiatric facility in a neighbouring city, staying once for eight weeks and a second time for ten. "(That's when) it really hit me, 'My God, I'm in a psychiatric hospital!' I could not believe that my path in life had brought me to that point." Yet in the psych hospital, she met people on a similar path, people who'd been defined as mentally ill but who had "a lot to offer."

Ever the performer, Hay would sometimes gather four chairs and play all the characters in an Alanis Morrissette video, jumping from chair to chair to draw a laugh or two. And sometimes, when they were feeling better, members of her in-patient audience would give her little presents in appreciation. Hay started thinking about what it was they all had in common. "Everyone was suffering and simply wanted to feel better. Still, we knew we had a stigma attached to us. We knew the visions people would get on the 'outside' if we told them we were in a psychiatric hospital. . . . But deep down inside, you are still you. It may be lost for a while, but you are there, and you have to continue moving forward."

For Hay, moving forward meant reporting for teacher's college just two weeks after that second long hospital stay. She'd already deferred her enrollment for a year, so this was her last chance. Although still depressed, she figured she'd better try. On her first day of classes, she managed a smile, thinking, "If only people knew." But no one did. No one seemed to notice anything.

That year at school was a struggle. She was still not well and took a lot of days off. In spite of that, she graduated on schedule. Right after graduation, she started the full-time teaching job she still holds today.

"The hardest thing about recovery," she now says, "is understanding that it's up to you to take responsibility for yourself. When you feel so bad mentally and physically, the last thing you want to do is take responsibility. I wanted to cut myself and wait for everyone else to figure out my life."

Four years have now passed since Joan Hay was last "officially" mentally ill. In that time she has, with the guidance of her therapist, figured out why she drank and why she cut herself, so that she no longer needs either of these forms of release. She has, with great difficulty, weaned herself off all but one of her medications. She still considers herself to be in recovery.

To the outside world that once seemed so very foreign to her, Joan Hay is today just one of the many hard-working, tax-paying citizens of a prosperous, mid-sized Canadian city. And yet, because of where she's been and everything she's overcome, she still faces possible rejection. She still struggles, in other words, with stigma, both self-imposed and not.

She does not, for example, date much. She doesn't trust the response she'd get if she said, "I actually spent two terms in a *psychiatric* hospital" (she's hamming it up). "I wouldn't present it quite that way, but that's basically what it comes down to. Will that person accept that? Or will they run screaming? . . . That's something I've been struggling through. I don't see myself as acceptable. Damaged goods, maybe. . . . I've avoided that part of my life, definitely, because I don't know how to deal with it yet." Call it anticipated stigma.

Then there's something you could think of as implied stigma, which can come from places you'd least expect. Doctors, for example, were quick to start Joan on all sorts of medications, but have been less willing to help her try stopping them. "[They said] I'm someone who's chronically, clinically – whatever c-word you want to put in there – depressed, and I will be the rest of my life. . . . And that this is the best that it's going to get. This is it. Your life can't get any better. I'm lucky to be at the level I am, out of the depths that I've come."

In the end, with as much research as she could find, she gradually worked herself off two drugs.* But there were withdrawal symptoms; she couldn't keep food down and lost fifteen pounds. She says her GP kept telling her the symptoms were all in her head. "She was very patronizing: 'You know your history and you get excited about things.' I thought I had run into all types of prejudices and stigma, but this was a new one."

But the most troubling examples of stigma – the ones she battles each day – happen on the job. Work has helped with her recovery, creating desperately needed structure and a certain awareness that other people are relying on her. "It's good to have the job; I know people who have floundered because they don't have a job to go to, so I'm grateful for that," she says. "It has pushed me in my recovery. I've forced myself to work, knowing once I get there it still may be tough, but at the end of the day I can say I've accomplished something. . . . On the other hand, when I've been ill, work has felt like my biggest enemy – the dark cloud. So many people depending on me, so many responsibilities, so overwhelming."

"I don't want people thinking that if I screw up it must be because I'm depressed or on a new med."

Every person who's been through the mental health system struggles with the question of who to tell, especially in the workplace. Joan, like many people, has even skirted her company health plan, despite its guarantees of privacy, and paid for her own psychotropic drugs to avoid any kind of paper trail. She has shared her history with her principal and vice-principal as well as three teachers she considers friends. "No one really knows the huge history," she explains, "but they know

---

* Before considering stopping any medication, please consult your doctor.

that I've been through a rough time, and I'm on meds and off meds and going through different things."

The responses have varied. Her bosses have been supportive, but there have also been examples of what can only be called overt stigma, such as the time a fellow teacher – one of those friends she'd told – lashed out at Joan after a work-related disagreement. "In front of the principal, she said that I needed a lobotomy," Joan relates. Another time, "She yelled down the hall, with the kids there, 'You know, you've got some *serious problems.*' I just walked away, but it stung me deeply, because you're going for my Achilles heel now. And for some reason I just feel that my Achilles heel is hanging out there all the time."

Hay senses that her colleagues believe she can't handle pressure well, that she's somehow too fragile. "I'm not viewed as solid. I could melt at any time. I've heard a few times, 'You've got to be careful with Joan.' And the reality of that, ironically, is that I probably have gone through more than they have. . . . I've gone through *so* much, and I'm still standing."

She worries she's judged more by what people assume she cannot do than by what she definitely *can* do. "I can spot a kid who has an emotional problem, who's depressed, who's manic, who's suicidal," she says. "I'm just so aware of mental health issues." Many of the children she teaches have emotional or behavioural problems, and they seem to know implicitly that with her, they won't be judged. "They have told me that they're cutting, that they're not eating, that they're depressed, that they're bipolar. . . . I'm just their sounding board, because I do know where they're coming from."

And she knows, by what she herself has been through, how to help. One girl, now in Grade 11, had done battle with Joan in the classroom for three years. "This kid *hated* me. This kid *threw* things at me. But I gave her boundaries. I told her when she was being a brat. When she was great, I told her she was. I told her she was really smart." Last year, when this girl returned from March break, she brought back a gift for Joan. It's a Mardi Gras necklace. "I'll keep that gift forever," Joan says, still moved. "I can't believe it's the same girl."

Joan Hay has recently convinced school management to set up a "mental health room" for students who need sympathetic listening and links to community outreach programs. She knows that for kids to feel okay about using the room, both teachers and students will have to be educated about stigma.

WISE WORDS ON STIGMA

"Stigma erodes confidence that mental disorders are valid, treatable health conditions. It leads people to avoid socializing, employing or working with, or renting to or living near persons who have a mental disorder. . . . Stigma tragically deprives people of their dignity and interferes with their full participation in society. It must be overcome."

— U.S. Surgeon General

"Today, stigma against those with psychiatric illness and those who treat them is the single most destructive element impeding progress in the care of the mentally ill. The effects of stigma begin with the hesitation of a person with mental illness to seek early psychiatric intervention. . . . I think of the Ethiopian proverb 'He who conceals his disease cannot expect to overcome it.' . . . We have all treated patients who ached needlessly and whose illnesses worsened because they felt anxious about, or disgraced by, their symptoms."

— Dr. Michael Myers, in a speech marking the end of his tenure, in 2001, as president of the Canadian Psychiatric Association

"Sadly, the most frequent contact the general public has with mental illness is through the media where, often, mental patients are depicted as unpredictable, violent and dangerous. . . . Such depictions stem from sensational reporting of crimes purportedly committed by a person with a mental illness, or from movies in which a popular plot, long exploited by the cinematographic industry, is that of the 'psychokiller.'"

— Dr. Julio Arboleda-Flórez, head of the department of psychiatry at Queen's University

DR. GRAEME CUNNINGHAM
On Self-Help Groups

He's a patient Dr. Graeme Cunningham will never forget.

His name was Rick,* and he walked in for an appointment on an otherwise ordinary day looking jaundiced and bloated and unusually unwell. Blood work confirmed what Cunningham already suspected: liver damage. He called him back to discuss the results.

"I said, 'You know, you've got cirrhosis. How's your drinking?' And he said, 'Pretty heavy.' And I said, 'You've got to quit,' thinking to myself, *You poor bastard*."

The pity he felt wasn't due to his patient's condition. It was because this unfortunate man would not be able to drink anymore. *Poor, unlucky fellow*, Cunningham was thinking. *How horrible and empty and pitiful his life will be without alcohol.*

Sobriety was something the physician could not imagine. Because the good doctor, you see, had himself been struggling with alcohol for years. He was also in serious denial – just like his father had been.

"My father was a family doctor, and he would drink a bottle of gin a day for almost as long as I can remember. And between the mid-1950s and his death in 1975, he never really drew a sober breath," says Cunningham, speaking with a crisp Scottish accent that more than three decades in Canada has softened only slightly.

Not only was his father alcoholic, but the disease made him violent, abusive, and unpredictable, capable of erupting at any time and for any reason. Sometimes he'd lash out against his wife, using words or fists, or a withering combination of both. On other occasions, the children, including Graeme, would be the target of his fury. It was not a healthy household.

"The message I got there was: 'Don't talk, don't trust, don't love, don't share, don't even necessarily be honest if it doesn't suit you. If you want something, get it – be violent. It's absolutely okay to punch, it's absolutely okay to kick, it's okay to beat people up.' That was the

---

* The name Rick is a pseudonym.

message, which resulted in [my becoming] someone who was aggressive and competitive, but felt inferior, if that makes any sense."

He also felt frustrated, seeing the connection between the booze and the constant mess at home. For a time, young Graeme would try to fix things by finding the bottles his father had stashed around the home. He'd pour the contents down the sink, again and again, hoping it would somehow make the problem go away. It never worked. There would always be more gin – or more punishment for having emptied a needed bottle.

Given his distaste for his father's behaviour, one might think Graeme would have steered clear of alcohol in any form. Problem is, addictions are so powerful and mystifying that they defy logic. Between genetics (several other male relatives drank heavily, suggesting the tendency was inherited), and the environment (chaotic and violent), Cunningham was at far greater risk than the average person for developing an addiction.

At least that's what the science tells us now. Back when Graeme was sixteen, however, almost nothing was known about this complex field. But he certainly remembers – with crystalline clarity – the night he took his first drink. He'd found something so extraordinary that he recounts it, some forty years later, with almost cinematic detail.

"I was sixteen. The girl's name was Brenda, as I recall. She had a cap on the right front upper tooth. It was about twenty to ten at night, the carpet was blue, the wallpaper was pale blue with little pink flowers on it. The tray was on top of the piano, which was a baby grand. It had a thistle emblem on it. There were five crystal glasses, and it was Johnny Walker Red Label.

"I took that stuff, and at that moment in time my intellect said, 'This is the stuff that makes your old man the way he is. This is not smart, Graeme.' But I thought, 'Well, shit, I'm going to try it anyway.' So I took it. And I was the only one at the party drinking. And I'll never forget the sense of, all of a sudden, feeling what I thought was *normal*. I still don't know what normal is, but my insides felt like your outsides looked. So you look put-together, you look relaxed, you look confident. Whereas I usually felt a mess in here.

"And I took that Scotch, I drank too much, I got sick, I went home, I threw up, I went to bed, I got up the next morning with a hangover. I'm still waiting for my mother to say, 'How come you came home drunk last night?' She hasn't said it yet, maybe she will, I don't know. But the memory of that reward was there. I've never ever had it that powerful since. The moment of that reward – it was profound. It was life-changing."

During his early years of what he now knows was alcoholism, Graeme would drink what he calls "peer-appropriately," meaning on Friday night you'd have a few beers with the boys and on Saturday nights – the big night out in Scotland – you'd get shit-faced. Sometimes it would be with his rugby pals, sometimes his fellow med students. No one suspected he had a problem, because he was simply treating alcohol the way his mates did. With one difference.

"The med students I was hanging out with were drinking heavily, too. What I didn't realize was that, when we became interns, they all stopped. But I continued. When I had a day off and I had some money, I drank to intoxication."

When Cunningham immigrated to Canada and eventually began practice in Central and Northern Ontario, money was no problem. Medicare ensured that a big fat cheque arrived regularly. Now he could afford to buy as much alcohol as he desired, and all the good brands, too. He'd have martinis after work, wine with supper, followed by a warming and generous concoction of Scotch and Drambuie. Typically, he'd down the equivalent of twenty-six ounces of liquor in an evening, sometimes more, becoming "quietly pissed" pretty much every night except for those when he was on call.

"So I'd go from someone who was apparently okay at five o'clock to a gibbering idiot by nine-thirty. That's what drove my family crazy. They just watched this deterioration in front of their eyes."

They also watched him attempt to conceal the behaviour. Efforts that made perfect, alcoholic sense to the successful doctor.

"I became a wine connoisseur; I joined the Opimian Society. I bought cases of wine, and they give you advice about laying it down for a month or six months until it matures. Well, I've discovered, from my perspective, that a wine connoisseur is simply a wino with a chequebook. And I drank a lot of pink, frothy, immature wine, because I just couldn't let it lay."

His first wife, with whom Cunningham says he often drank (and with whom he had two children), left him in the early 1970s for another man. The breakup fed into Graeme's belief that, at his core, he was not a good person. The fact he had an excellent and growing reputation in medicine (he didn't drink on the job in those days) was irrelevant.

"By this time, I had what I call my voice. And my voice goes something like this: I'd get an award, or I'd get a title, or I'd get a position of authority, like Chief Resident, Medicine, and on the outside people would be saying, 'Good for you. Well done.' And my voice would say, '*If you only knew me. If you only knew the things that I was doing and the person that I was becoming you'd never speak to me again and you would leave.*'

"So there was an inside feeling of not being good enough. I was a fake, I was inadequate. Do you get the sense of egomania with an inferiority complex? The arrogant doctor who doesn't like himself? And the arrogance is a front. A front of fear. And so, at times, it was impossible to stay in my own skin. So I continued to drink. And I moved from the point of enjoying alcohol to the point of actually needing it to feel, to survive, just to get by."

Though unaware of it, Cunningham was now making the transition from someone society might call "a heavy drinker" to a person who was out of control, whose entire life – ranging from his social choices through to his career decisions – began to revolve around the use of alcohol. The doctor sought out appointments to numerous medical bodies and committees. The frequent meetings in Toronto meant he'd be put up in a plush hotel and have a good opportunity to get smashed, either in his room or at a bar where nobody knew him.

Similarly, Cunningham avoided situations where the booze couldn't flow freely. If a friend who did not drink heavily extended an invite to the cottage for the weekend, the thought of not getting his hands on enough alcohol would send the doctor into a panic so great he would automatically decline.

"The choices were all to allow me to drink more, in secret, because of shame and because of fear of discovery," he says. "So my repertoire in life, my options, were narrowing."

He learned little tricks along the way, ones that his father had no doubt discovered decades earlier. A flat or square bottle, for example, works much better in the car than round bottles, which have a tendency to roll out from the under the seat. He learned that office samples of "Vitamin V" – Valium – would help take the edge off when he needed a drink at work. He learned that the police in his small Northern city generally took drunken doctors home when they'd been driving instead of to jail. All this while raising two children from his first marriage.

When he remarried (to a woman who immediately pegged him as an alcoholic but loved him nonetheless), his wife soon gave birth to twins. Cunningham now looks back in horror to a night when wife Linda was out and he was putting fresh diapers on his infant son, who was perched on a change table. Seriously impaired, Cunningham lost his balance, pulling the table over as he fell backwards. The child went tumbling through the air, but he managed – just barely – to catch him.

"He could have been badly injured; he was just a little baby. But I was drunk."

Despite everything, he still believed he was nothing like his father. The mistake was in not realizing that his father had more than twenty extra years of alcoholism under his belt. In reality, Cunningham was already on the same path – he just couldn't see where it was leading.

"In the context of this illness, the first thing you lose and the last thing you get back is insight. I mean, you'd look at me and say, 'Geez, Graeme, do you not *see* what you're doing?' And I really wouldn't."

And then one day, who should make a return visit to the office? Pathetic old Rick. It had been about a month since Cunningham had sent him on his way, shaking his head at the poor bastard's misfortune.

Except *this* Rick looked great. He was wearing a suit, his belly was flat, the jaundice was gone, his eyes crystal-clear. The man who had walked out of the office so wretched and miserable now looked reborn. Rick had got his job back, his family life, and he wasn't drinking.

There was something, well, *attractive* about what Rick now had; Cunningham asked him how he'd managed to achieve it.

"I'm staying sober, doc, in a program called Alcoholics Anonymous." On some level, Graeme knew that he needed help, so he decided to sit in on a few AA meetings himself. They scared the hell out of him.

"The honesty threatened me. The out-and-out just straight sharing was beyond me. I would drink before I went, drink after I left. So it didn't work."

But the seed had been sown. Over time, as Cunningham's alcoholism progressed, when it finally, inevitably, began to show itself at work (he started drinking vodka on the job), he had an epiphany. While at the hospital, he had a sudden and clear revelation that if he continued drinking, he would die. So shattering and pure was this insight that a very shaken alcoholic went home and immediately poured a drink to cope.

"I was sitting in my basement. It was ten o'clock at night, it was a Friday, third of January, 1986, in Timmins, ass-deep in snow outside, thirty below, and a voice said, literally, in my ear, 'I'm staying sober, doc, in a program called Alcoholics Anonymous.' I'll never forget that. Rick was literally sitting right beside me. He wasn't, but that's what I heard. It was his voice, as clear as I'm sitting here."

Cunningham picked up the phone and called the local AA line. Someone immediately answered. Cunningham gave his address. Some thirty seconds later – and he's not kidding – there was a knock on his door. The person manning the AA phone that night lived just three doors down the street.

After a "Timmins treatment" (a few days drinking coffee and puking into a bucket in his neighbour's basement while AA stalwarts told him their own stories), Dr. Cunningham was on his way to an alcohol rehab in Toronto. He knocked back what booze he could on the plane, got to the facility, and was sitting in a chair thinking how absolutely wretched and defeated and weak he felt.

He'd just come off a drunk. His breath was sour, his face unshaven, his hands shaking. He was also feeling deeply, deeply ashamed.

Just then a pleasant woman came up and put her hand on his shoulder. She introduced herself as Anne,* said she'd been there ten days and that she'd show him around. Cunningham told her how awful he felt.

"'Yes, I know, it's rough on the first day or two,'" she replied.

"I said: 'But I should *know* better.'

"'Why?'

"'Because I'm a *doctor*.'

"And she said, 'So am I.'"

Cunningham never drank again. His personal, professional, and spiritual growth in the coming years would lead to his becoming the director of the addiction division at the Homewood Health Centre in Guelph and an associate professor of psychiatry at McMaster University. It would also lead to his learning that his own recovery depended on sharing the possibilities of sobriety with others. Depended on *helping*.

"To keep it, I've got to give it away. To keep my sobriety, to keep my recovery, I have to give it away. That's moving from that place of infantile omnipotence, when I was sick and feeling I was the centre of the world and the world owed me, to a place – and I'm using psychiatry and psychology jargon – of altruistic service, where I can be of service to my fellow person without reservation. In other words, I'd look at a heroin addict and I don't care who they are, what they've done, where they've come from; I'm just glad they're here, and ask myself what can I do to help them change."

Anne did not fare as well.

"I saw Anne's obituary in the *Canadian Medical Journal* two years ago. Died of alcoholism. Lost her licence, lost her kids, including her twins, lost everything. Died in the street, a bag lady. I don't know why I'm here now, sober, but that woman reached out to me that night and said, 'It's okay to be a sick doc.' And, God, I needed to hear that."

In the ultimate scheme of things, Anne may well have contributed to a far greater good. The program at the Homewood, with Cunningham

---

* The name Anne is a pseudonym.

in charge, has now successfully treated several thousand addicted health professionals, ranging from doctors and nurses and dentists through to veterinarians and pharmacists.

In addition, Dr. Graeme Cunningham helped develop a province-wide program where physicians or their spouses can call an 800 number in total confidence and begin that often daunting search for help. Cunningham calls it the best in the country.

"I'm very proud of that. I don't mean that in an egotistical sense.

"And I sometimes think of my dad looking down and saying, 'Good job, son.'"

WISE WORDS

This pithy little parable comes from the hit TV show *The West Wing*. Leo, the White House chief of staff (and a recovering alcoholic), offers it up to Josh, who is struggling with posttraumatic stress disorder after being shot. It speaks to the value of all self-help movements.

"A man is walking down the street, and he falls down a hole. He yells for help. A doctor walks by, sees the man, writes a prescription, throws it down into the hole, and keeps walking. Later, a priest walks by, sees the man, writes down a prayer, throws it in the hole, and keeps walking. Then a friend walks by, sees the man, and jumps down the hole with him. The man says, 'What did you do that for? Now we're both stuck.' The friend replies, 'Yeah, but I've been down here before, and I know the way out.'"

SELF HELP

Research has consistently shown that self-help programs are good for our mental health, increasing self-esteem and coping skills, while reducing hospitalizations. Self-help groups can be found in every part of the country and for virtually every diagnosis. Some names and numbers are listed in the appendix of *The Last Taboo*.

LINKING DRINKING

▶ Substance abuse and substance dependence are listed as psychiatric disorders in the diagnostic manuals used by psychiatrists.

▶ About *half* of patients with serious mental disorders develop alcohol or other substance abuse problems (U.S. Surgeon General's report).

▶ The same U.S. report notes that in any given year, about 3 per cent of the population will have both a mental disorder and an addictive disorder. Another 6 per cent have only addictive disorders.

▶ The link between substance disorders and mental disorders works both ways. In a six-year follow-up study in the United States (by the National Institute of Mental Health), 28 per cent of people who started out with alcoholism and 35 per cent of those starting out with a drug-use disorder had developed major depression at follow-up.

▶ Men are more likely than women to drink every day and to engage in hazardous or harmful drinking (Centre for Addiction and Mental Health).

▶ Substance use and abuse tends to increase with income level (Centre for Addiction and Mental Health).

BARB AND DARRYL HALEY
On Becoming Advocates

Luke was the imp, the little charmer with the huge brown eyes and wide smile beneath that flop of blond hair. Here was a kid who bowled people over with the sheer force of his enthusiasms. He wore, quite literally, his passions on his sleeve, once cheering on his favourite baseball team at the SkyDome by wearing Blue Jays pants, shirt, hat, socks, *and* underwear. Ten-year-old "Lukie" was named Second Fan of the Day, his face flashing on the giant JumboTron for the entire stadium to see. But even that wasn't good enough; he said afterwards that if only he'd flashed his Jays underwear, he might've been named *First* Fan.

Ben was the big brother of the family, all red hair and freckles and long limbs. Towering over his classmates, he seemed older than his years. Ben was the romantic, the "artsy-fartsy" teenager who wrote poetry and opined at length on any subject. "He was headstrong," his mother says. "When he was three, I can remember saying to him, 'This is *not* the United Nations – we are not negotiating this!'"

Barbara Haley pauses for a moment, remembering. "They were fun," she says quietly. "They were really fun. And I will miss that forever."

In her sunny living room, she spreads out photographs of Ben and Luke in various smiling poses. Her husband, Darryl, is down in the basement looking for other family mementoes. Perhaps he also needs a quiet moment to himself after a long and draining afternoon spent answering questions.

Although this chapter is about recovery, there really is no such thing for Barbara and Darryl Haley. When your only two children – your Luke and your Ben – have died of suicide, recovery is not within the realm of possibilities. All that remains is survival and the need to find some purpose, some reason to carry on. Which the Haleys have been doing, every day since their sons' deaths.

"Somebody once asked me, 'How many hours can go by without you thinking of the children?'" says Barbara. "And I looked at him, and I said, '*Hours*? It's minutes.'"

She and Darryl have made it a personal mission to speak out, wherever possible, about kids and mental health, kids and suicide, kids and the need for better services. They educate and advocate – for more research, more facilities, more care. "The bottom line? I don't want to see other beautiful children die when they don't have to," Barbara says.

And every day, Barbara does something few of us think to do in our busy, scattered lives. She makes the effort to do something nice – a small gesture or kind word – for someone. Then she says to herself, "That one was for you, Luke" or "for you, Ben." She does this "to keep in mind who they were as people. Because they were kind people."

She remembers Luke, on a family trip to Washington, seeing homeless people for the first time. Emptying his last pennies into various outstretched hands, Luke cried at the thought of so much suffering.

And she remembers Ben, in ninth grade, working as a peer counsellor for younger children. After Ben died, some of those children
came to see Barb and Darryl. "They said, 'He was the one we could
talk to,'" Barbara says.

Perhaps this interview is one of Barbara's kind gestures, her daily
tribute to her boys. And, if so, then this story is for them: for Luke
and for Ben.

Seven years ago, on a warm spring day, Barbara Haley was lying on
the grass, watching her two boys play, and feeling blessed with everything the world had to offer.

By the following spring, both boys were gone.

Another jarring contrast, a photo kept tucked away because Barbara
cannot often bear to see it. In a silver frame etched with stars, there is
Luke in a wetsuit, hamming for the camera, an enormous grin on his
twelve-year-old face. "I mean, who would've thought?" Barbara says in
wonderment. "This was taken two days before he died."

How can such a thing happen? Every parent surely wonders. And
yet it *does* happen, in every kind of family, in every part of the country.
And sometimes even to the best of parents, in the best of all possible
worlds.

"It's so awful, suicide. It takes a toll on everybody. You feel like
you're so rejected," Barbara says. "And there's never an answer for it.
There's *never* an answer."

"There is no closure," Darryl adds.

The Haley boys grew up in the picturesque and prosperous community of St. Margarets Bay, Nova Scotia, an idyllic kind of place
where the houses are grand and the backyard is the ocean. Summer
weekends were spent sailing and motorboating in the Bay.

Luke was an athletic boy, an excellent swimmer and skier. But by
the age of ten, he had started experiencing migraine headaches. He'd
also had a hard time learning to read. And the summer he turned
twelve, his mother noticed a dip in his self-esteem. "I actually had
thought, 'I'm going to watch this,'" Barbara says. "And I actually
had given myself a deadline and said, 'If this isn't any better, if he

doesn't even out over the summer, then we're off to the family doctor.' "

The Haleys had already consulted with doctors over Luke's reading troubles, his migraines, and also some stomach pains. "And each time I said, 'Do you think he needs to talk to somebody?' " Barbara recalls. "And I think what happened is, because you look like a mother who is saying the right things, because you're saying . . . 'I'm not feeling quite right about this,' because you have actually come in and said that, [the reaction is] 'Oh no, you're looking after it; you're fine.' " In fact, Barbara *does* look like the quintessential caring mother, with her kind face and welcoming manner. She teaches special education; Darryl Haley is a chartered accountant and business consultant.

Around this time, one of Luke's young friends died, in a probable suicide, at the age of ten. Both Ben and Luke attended the funeral, because they wanted to, and both came away profoundly affected. "One of them threw up in the car afterwards," Barbara says. "There was a lot of crying."

That June, Luke turned twelve. And in early July, Ben and Luke's uncle, Barbara's brother-in-law, died of cancer. Barb and Darryl were uncertain about putting the boys through the emotional strain of another funeral. "So we talked it over with them, and they said, 'I think our uncle would like us to stay here and do our sailing lessons,' " Barbara says.

She takes a deep breath and then continues. "So we left to go to this funeral, and Luke hanged himself while we were away. And his brother found him. Ben found him. And Ben, because they'd had a little spat prior to that – nothing out of the ordinary – blamed himself. Ben always blamed himself." Barbara pauses, takes another breath. "The only thing I could think of at the airport was: I didn't have to see him. And Ben did."

While Barbara and Darryl made their way back home, friends, neighbours, and clergy immediately offered their support. The RCMP came to the house in plain clothes, and repeatedly told Ben he'd done nothing wrong.

"That summer, he didn't do too badly," Barbara says. But in the fall, his teachers began commenting that he seemed distant – well-behaved but not really paying attention in class. Several teachers, knowing what had happened, rallied around him; the art teacher, the music teacher "hauled that kid through, and we got a couple of extra months with him because of those people."

The Haleys arranged for Ben to see a psychiatrist every week (no mean feat considering the waiting lists for child psychiatrists). And he liked this doctor very much.

His friends were also incredibly supportive, even waiting outside the psychiatrist's office for Ben's appointments to finish, just to make sure he was okay.

But that winter, despite all the support, Ben was not okay. In fact, he was becoming more and more depressed. "By January, he was changing. And we both knew in January something very awful was happening," Barb says. "We could progressively see him go downhill. The hair started turning different colours. Nails started turning different colours."

"He really got into heavy metal music in a big, big way," Darryl says. "And he painted the inside of his room completely black. . . . And when [the popular grunge-rock singer] Curt Cobain died, that was it. Cobain died [of suicide] in April. And from April to August, it was *bad*."

That spring, Ben attended the senior prom. He was only in the tenth grade, but a twelfth-grader had asked him to be her date for the evening. Barbara escorted them to a park to take photographs. By then, Ben was so clearly unwell that she remembers thinking, " 'I'm not going to be taking his picture again.' Somehow I had the feeling that what he was doing was giving himself significant moments – i.e., the prom and things like that – and he was fighting it, but he was on his way out."

Ben said he found it difficult to be around the house, that he'd look at his parents and feel responsible for his brother's death. "I can remember holding him, and telling him we loved him, and we didn't blame him. . . . And I could understand why it would be so difficult to come home."

"In retrospect," Darryl adds, "what we should've done was just packed up and gone."

"It was like a Jenga game or something," Barbara says, "where the pieces were being hauled out of him and you were just hoping that you could either push them in or hold them up or give him a wall, or give him some time. It was awful. It was just awful."

In July, Ben was admitted to a Halifax hospital, to one of a very limited number of beds then set aside for adolescents with mental illnesses. He was placed on the children's psychiatric ward, Ward Four-South, and assigned a bed more than a foot shorter than he was. (Ben, now sixteen, was more than six feet tall.) His roommate was a twelve-year-old boy whose condition was deemed so fragile that Ben was not allowed to be in the room during the daytime.

"So basically," Darryl says, angrily, "what they gave him was a short bed to sleep in at night. Otherwise he had to be out of the room."

Ben was assessed by a psychiatric team which, recognizing the setting was less than ideal, recommended he be released. After three days on the ward, they sent him home.

"I had serious problems with that," Darryl asserts. "I knew my son was *not well*. And I stated that if they released him they did so over my objection. And they released him. And ten days later, he was dead."

"I had gone out to tutor a student," Barbara says. "And we came back and we found him."

One year, one month, and one day after his brother had died, Ben shot himself. He left a note for his parents, saying that he loved them, and please not to blame themselves, but he was very, very tired.

"Tired of fighting the depression and of pretending things were okay in front of people when they weren't," Barbara says. "His last words were, 'I love you Mom and Dad. Carry on.'"

A few years later, Barbara would say these words aloud, on television, for a documentary about teen suicide. She shared the details of the note, and of Ben's death, with a local CBC reporter. She described the day, scarcely a year earlier, in which she'd thought the world was perfect.

It was one way to carry on, to do as her son had urged.

After Ben's death, Barb and Darryl Haley did pack up and leave St. Margarets Bay. They moved to nearby Halifax, where they now live in a large, elegant Victorian house they share with a big tomcat named Julius, who purrs on Barbara's lap and tugs at the microphone cord with a massive paw while she talks. The lanky, red-haired cat wandered into their home one day and decided to stay, and Barbara was struck by his resemblance to lanky, red-haired Ben. "Do you think he's in there?" she asks, and smiles.

You'd be surprised to know that Barbara and Darryl do smile, and laugh, quite often. Humour helps them through the "black hole" of grief and depression.

"I had never had such pain. Such *pain*," Barb says. "And that is hard to explain to somebody who hasn't been there: that it's profound, it's 100 per cent, it's overwhelming, and it's there."

"It's all-pervasive," Darryl says. "It's just black. And you just keep working at putting one foot in front of the other."

What inspires that foot to move is pretty much the same as what keeps most of us going through those most difficult times in life. Family, friends, religious faith. Although Barb admits with a small laugh, "I haven't been back to church. I still have a little thing about God. I'm still a little mad. And I figure He can take it."

Although many a marriage has dissolved in grief, theirs has been a source of strength, and sometimes in unexpected ways. "Particularly during the first couple of years," Darryl says, "we cycled completely differently, almost 180 degrees, which was good. When Barb was down, I was up. When I was down, she was up."

Barb looks towards her husband. "And one of the things that we really said was that we weren't going to lose each other, too. We're just not going to let that happen. And in the sickest of moments, we had this agreement that one was not going to leave the other one alone."

"If we were going to go," Darryl explains, "we were going to go together."

"And so we had this place picked out," Barb continues. "Up the Mersey Road. You know, one of those backwoods roads. And we'd kind of look at each other sometimes and say, 'Well, are you ready to go up to the Mersey?'"

They both laugh at that, at themselves.

Barb and Darryl say that time does not heal and grief does not abate. What happens instead is that "you do gain the ability to divert yourself," Darryl says. "You learn that."

Immediately after Ben's death, the Haleys focused on his friends. Sometimes a suicide can trigger more suicides in vulnerable people close to the first victim – a phenomenon known as cluster suicides. The Haleys were aware of this possibility. And in fact, there was another suicide at Ben's high school soon after his death. The Haleys immediately started working with the local hospital, school, and clergy to set up intervention sessions for the students. They've been active advocates ever since.

"It started initially to help them [Ben's schoolmates], to get information to their families, to get information to the school, to get these children watched, to get them cared for," Barb explains. "That was sort of the focus for the first two years."

As they started to volunteer their services, they heard from other parents upset with the mental health system: with too few informed doctors, shortages of child psychiatrists, and eternally long waiting lists. The turning point came when they picked up a newspaper and read that hospital psychiatric services for youths were being moved to a former cafeteria space, "a hole," Barbara says, next to the smoker's lounge with thin walls and little privacy. "Talk about marginalizing of services, and kids. And that just did it for me."

"It just seemed that there was a need for somebody to stand up from the community and say, 'Hey, we value this service, and it's necessary,'" Darryl says.

The problem was, few parents were willing to stand up and be heard; stigma, the fear of being judged or shamed, kept them quiet. The Haleys, meanwhile, felt they had nothing left to lose. "Who better to speak up?" Barbara says. "What could we possibly lose? We'd seen the worst, so actually we were in the best position to speak out. Nobody could do anything to us that could hurt us any more."

In 1997, the Haleys sat down with representatives from the Dalhousie University medical school and IWK Grace Health Centre, the largest hospital in Halifax. Together, they agreed to establish a research chair in adolescent mental health. "Here was something we could do," Darryl says, "which was to establish a chair, which would act as a lightning rod. And it's there forever."

First, they had to raise some $2 million. Initially, the fundraising was tough; corporations were reluctant to get behind such an "unsexy" issue. (One marketing executive went so far as to say, "We couldn't be seen to be supporting a cause like that!") So the team set out to raise their own profile. In 1999, they organized an international symposium on adolescent mental health with an A-list of speakers and an attendance of more than 400. In 2000, the group started an annual "Reaching Out Run," with school teams attracting sponsors from across Nova Scotia.

In 2001, they finally met their goal, having raised $1.3 million from various donors, and a full $1 million from Sun Life Financial. The research chair became the first of its kind in North America.

"Our thought was, okay, we get the chair. It will be a point of excellence, it will bring intelligent researchers and professionals, it will help make us a centre of excellence, and, when that happens, then you get the spin-off effects, so that you get the lobbying to government, you get best practices to patients. This is our goal," says Barbara.

The Haleys say that services have already begun to improve in their city. IWK Grace has set up a mental health clinic, with private funding, to help junior-high students and their families. "They created a network for those kids that wasn't there before," Darryl says tearfully.

As Darryl has done for her several times during the interview, Barbara now steps in to continue her husband's thought. "That's right, it wasn't there," she says gently. "Is that the purpose of my children dying? No, that's not it. But I think as people – just as people – we both felt we couldn't see our children's friends die. We couldn't see our children's friends' parents go through that. You just couldn't stand by. You had to act, you just had to. There just wasn't any choice."

What's helped the Haleys most of all are those friends of Luke and Ben. There were times, the Haleys say, when they thought they'd completely lost it, and then this group of kids would come knocking on their door. "Boy, did they ever pull us through," Barb says.

That first Halloween, as the Haleys handed out candy at the door, a crew of them showed up looking for costumes. "You guys always had the dress-up box," they said. "So we dressed them up, and they went out trick-or-treating, and nobody felt great but everybody felt better," Barbara says.

On prom night – the night that Ben would have graduated – they appeared in their ball gowns and snazzy suits so that the Haley backyard was once again filled with young people.

In a touching tribute to Ben, one of his schoolmates – she had sat beside him in tenth-grade art class – prepared a radio documentary about the Haley family. She spoke to Barb and Darryl, and to Ben's closest friends.

At one point in the documentary, a young male voice explains the connection he feels to Ben's parents, saying "When I'm with them, I still feel that I can be close to Ben. But by the same token, they're role models to me; they're very smart, successful people, and I just enjoy their company, and I like being with them."

Next, a young female voice, another friend of Ben's, says, "I think that they are a gift to all of us. . . . They are so intelligent and worldly and funny and amusing and entertaining and up for anything and welcoming. I mean, who doesn't know the security code to their house?"

Then Barbara's voice, overrun with emotion, saying, "There could have been a lot of judging of who we were as parents, and who we are as people, and what our home was. And the fact that those kids . . . still wanted to be around our home, I think it helped us see that we tried to be good parents. . . . They'd come up and they'd hug us. And they'd say things like, I would *love* to have had you for my mom or dad."

Those kids are an integral part of why the Haleys do what they do, why they carry on. And why they continue to push for a better mental health system for young people. But Barbara says it best. "I'm looking at children like my Luke, my Ben, or it could've been Emily or the little kid across the street. . . . We have these talented, wonderful kids who have things to offer and give, as every human does, and they could cut their life off for want of a couple of thousand dollars worth of service? And they're not getting service because of stigma and prejudice. . . . And that's wrong. It is *wrong*."

By the end of the interview, the father who at first had seemed more angry than sad has shed tears, and the mother who had seemed more sad has voiced her anger. And at the end of this spring day, after the interview has been completed – a sacrifice that will take its toll for days to come – Barbara and Darryl Haley wait with their visitor for a cab. From their large front porch, we look out onto the street, a quiet street lined with tall trees and big front lawns that have finally turned to green with the first few warm days of the season. The street is quiet, save for the sound of the next-door neighbours' two boys playing basketball in their driveway. They leap enthusiastically towards the hoop, dodge from side to side. Like every teenage boy these days, their shirts are baggy and their feet seem huge. The Haleys wave and smile, and the boys echo back hellos. When Barb exclaims at the beautiful weather, they both smile politely before returning to their game. And we all sit quietly for a moment, listening to the familiar sound of a ball going *thump*, *thump*, *thump* against the pavement.

Barbara and Darryl Haley have, with a group of concerned people from their community, established a corporation called Reaching Out: Youth and Mental Health Inc. to raise awareness of youth mental health issues across the Maritimes, and eventually across the country. For more information, see their Web site: <www.reachingout.ca>.

ADOLESCENT SUICIDE

▶ In 1997, there were 312 reported suicides in Canada by people under the age of twenty. Almost 80 per cent of those suicides were by males (Statistics Canada).

▶ Canada's adolescent suicide rate has tripled since the 1950s, and, along with motor-vehicle accidents, is one of the leading causes of death among adolescents.

▶ More teenagers and young adults die of suicide than of cancer, heart disease, AIDS, pneumonia, influenza, birth defects, and stroke combined (Centre for Addiction and Mental Health).

YOUTH AND MENTAL HEALTH

▶ In a survey of almost 5,000 Ontario students (Grade 7 to high school graduates):
  • 30 per cent reported high levels of psychological distress
  • 13 per cent said they'd seen a health professional for mental health reasons in the preceding year

(*The Mental Health and Well-Being of Ontario Students Report*, Centre for Addiction and Mental Health)

▶ Approximately 20 per cent of children aged four to sixteen have a diagnosable psychiatric disorder that requires professional help. That means more than *1 million* Canadian children are currently living with identifiable disorders. A further 20 per cent experience some form of psychological disturbance.

▶ According to the U.S. Surgeon General's "Report on Mental Health," the best estimates for prevalence of mental disorder among children and adolescents are as follows:
  • Anxiety disorders – 13 per cent
  • Mood disorders – 6.2 per cent
  • Disruptive disorders – 10.3 per cent (e.g. conduct disorder, oppositional defiant disorder)

▶ Approximately 80 per cent of young people who need help for a mental illness receive no treatment.

―――ᴍᴍ―――

"A CALL TO ARMS: PART ONE"
by Don Tapscott

There is a pernicious notion that mental illness is somehow a flaw or failure in a person's character, rather than a treatable disease. As a society we pay a heavy price for this false perception.

I care a great deal about this issue. I began my career years ago as a psychometrist and later as a psychologist. But my interest is also personal.

Tony Blair's government in Britain has launched a campaign to overcome the stigma of mental illness. The theme is "Every Family." I know how apt this expression is. My brother Dave, two years my younger, became ill in the early 1970s. We'll never know the real diagnosis; at the time he was diagnosed with "drug-induced schizophrenia." I'm now told Dave may have suffered from a severe clinical depression.

Dave was a bright and kind person, a good student, a contract bridge master, and a talented pianist and oboe player. He was funny, fun to be with, and, with the rest of my family, we had many great times together. Despite early symptoms he graduated from Trent University, which was a good place for him because of its student-centred learning. He didn't get lost in the crowd there. But after a fifteen-year battle with the disease, he gave up, dying under circumstances that suggest suicide – in a single-vehicle accident on a deserted road late one night.

The Tapscott Chair in Schizophrenia Studies is named in Dave's memory and in honour of our parents, Don and Mary Tapscott, who worked tirelessly to keep Dave healthy. After he graduated, he was in and out of work, living for prolonged periods at my parents' house in the Ontario town of Orillia. They spent every day with him when he was there, playing bridge, talking, making music, following various sports teams, going to the lake together. My younger sister was still in school for some of this time and was close to Dave, but she was also very saddened and frightened by his illness. My parents read everything they could find about mental illness and its treatment and took Dave to treatment facilities, institutions, and doctors across the province.

For two years, Dave lived with me, my girlfriend Ana, and my two other brothers in a house we all shared in Toronto. I was travelling a lot, and it was often left to Ana to spend hours with Dave, trying to help and comfort him as best she could. The stress and sadness were punctuated by great times; for example, Ana and I married in the house, and Dave played piano at our wedding, beautifully as usual. We all remember it as a very happy time.

Assuming the diagnosis of schizophrenia was correct, Dave was a victim of one of the most devastating and costly illnesses of our time. Patients with schizophrenia occupy one of every twelve hospital beds in Canada, more than any other medical condition. Four of every ten with the disorder attempt suicide to escape its horrors. Most victims come from families with no history of the disease. People with this affliction have too little care and too little understanding.

It is instructive to turn the clock back and consider my brother's fate in earlier times. If Dave became psychotic circa 1900, he would have been placed in an asylum – likely the Toronto Lunatic Asylum – a horrific setting of chronic illness isolated from the mainstream of medicine and society. Treatment was not so much an exercise in medicine as an exercise in bricks and mortar. He would have spent his life there under nightmarish conditions. If he did not somehow recover spontaneously he would remain incarcerated for life.

My first job after graduating in psychology in 1970 was at a mental health centre for the so-called "criminally insane." I remember touring the basement rooms, essentially dungeons, complete with metal shackles on the walls to restrain and punish difficult patients. This was just thirty years ago.

Circa 1950, if Dave had been lucky, he could have gone to the tiny Toronto Psychiatric Hospital founded by Dr. C. K. Clarke. There was still little research into the biology of the brain as a cause of mental illness. While barbiturates were used widely to sedate patients, there were still no antipsychotic drugs. In the United States and Canada, the main focus of investigation and even treatment of mental illness was psychotherapy. In a wonderful book entitled *A History of Psychiatry*, Toronto's Dr. Edward Shorter writes that at mid-twentieth century, psychiatry became enraptured with the notion that psychological problems arose of unconscious conflicts over long past events, especially those of a sexual nature. For several decades, psychiatrists were glad to adopt this theory of illness, he writes, especially because it gave them an opportunity to get out of the asylum and into private practice, a better income, and a little social respect.

By 1970, when Dave became ill, science had overtaken Freud, and mental illness had returned to the fold of other medical specialties. Drug therapy was the treatment of choice for psychosis based on early systematic experimentation into the chemistry of the brain. But my brother wasn't a big beneficiary. After his first psychotic attacks, we tried to get him into the Clarke, but it was full. At eleven o'clock one winter night, he was taken by ambulance and police escort from our house in Toronto to a general hospital that was visited, infrequently, by psychiatric professionals. Various new medications were tried, but in hindsight the doses given him were likely five to ten times greater than necessary. Such overdoses caused terrible side effects for him, and so he didn't stick with them – classic non-compliance. As he told me one day, "When I'm off the drugs, I might feel crazy, but that's better than feeling pulverized." Some of these medications caused severe swelling of various parts of his body, dryness of his mouth and throat to the point where he could not speak, and ultimately complete immobility.

What if Dave were in his early twenties and became ill today? Things would be very different. If he were fortunate to live in a handful of Canadian cities such as Halifax, London, or Calgary, he would be admitted into the first-episode clinic of a psychiatric hospital. In Toronto, where Dave lived, this would be the Centre for Addiction and Mental Health.

A multi-disciplinary team of medical, psychiatric, and psychological personnel would conduct an extensive evaluation into the nature and causes of his illness. For starters, his diagnosis would much more likely be correct. Schizophrenia? Perhaps. Or was he a victim of depression, which can cause psychosis? Was he psychotic because of his use of amphetamines, which have been found to increase the action of dopamine and destabilize brain chemistry? A correct diagnosis would enable the development of an optimal treatment plan without so much of the trial-and-error treatment of the seventies.

A second multi-disciplinary team consisting of medical, social work, and occupational therapy professionals would meet his needs and orchestrate his integration back into the community. In the 1970s, "community integration" meant sending people to the street or to unsupported families who had little chance of coping with the illness. Today, there is a much greater appreciation that people need to be engaged on their own terms and treated in a comprehensive way that meets their complete individual needs.

But even this 2002 scenario – available to only a small proportion of Canadians – pales in comparison to the improvements being made in the treatment of other diseases.

According to Dr. Mary Seeman, a leading schizophrenia researcher, we have learned more about the brain in the last decade than in all of human history. I am optimistic we could make even greater progress in the next few years.

Some day in the not-too-distant future, the following scenario will occur. Dave would simply never have a first episode. His illness would be diagnosed and treated before it became manifest. For example, there is a theory that schizophrenia results from excessive elimination of nerve synapses (connections between nerve cells) during adolescence compared to the rate of elimination seen in healthy individuals. If this turned out to be true, then it might be possible to develop medications that slow this process down to a normal rate.

In another future scenario, the evaluation of a blood sample after birth could identify a genetic predisposition to brain disease or a vulnerability to amphetamine-induced psychosis or some other pathology, and an effective preventative treatment plan could be implemented. This might involve some kind of gene therapy by which some genes could be modified to ensure that some critical step in the development of schizophrenia does not take place. It might involve advising against exposure to particular forms of substance abuse.

Or, perhaps in his early teens, Dave's GP, or a teacher or parent, could identify pre-symptom evidence that he was having trouble coping, which we know today is often advance warning of the onset of illness. A preventative program could be implemented.

Dave would have a great shot at a happy and fulfilling life.

The future is not something to be predicted; it is something to be achieved. Such a bright future needs funding, and right now it's not getting it.

The question is, How come? Why has society been able to marshal the resources to attack other diseases but not those of the brain? To say the brain is more complicated is too easy. I believe we are paralyzed by an all-pervasive stigma that goes back centuries. We fear what we don't understand. And fear gets in the way of doing the right thing.

Don't we need a campaign to establish the understanding that depression, schizophrenia, and other mental disorders are treatable illnesses, not failings of character?

Perhaps the term "mental illness" is itself a misnomer, a throwback to the days when scientists thought there was a mind-body distinction. It was not Dave's mind that needed effective treatment, it was the bio-chemistry of his brain. He didn't need mental health; he needed a healthy brain, free from disease, no less than he needed a healthy heart. He did not have a failing of his mind, or personality, or character; he had a failing of his brain.

Let's decide to launch a campaign to end the stigma around illnesses of the brain and get real funding to end this human tragedy. There are so many brilliant investigators in Canada (psychiatrists, molecular biologists, epidemiologists, geneticists, pharmacologists) with the courage, curiosity, and commitment to tackle this issue. The brain is no longer viewed as the backwoods of medicine, but its forefront.

On October 9, 2000, the Nobel Prize in medicine was given to three brain researchers – two molecular biologists and a psychiatrist – for discoveries regarding the way in which disturbances in signals between nerve cells can give rise to neurological and psychiatric diseases. This work has already led to the development of important new drug treatments.

The widespread popularity of Prozac has begun to make it acceptable to discuss depression. Many people have begun to tell their personal stories and help change public perceptions. I cannot overstate how important these initiatives are. We need a sea change in the public perception of these illnesses. Let's stop whispering about mental health. Let's start talking loudly and often.

There is a role in these discussions for every individual and every institution in this country. Governments, businesses, community groups, unions, and not-for-profit groups should all participate. Governments at all levels need to provide the kind of leadership they have shown in mobilizing support to combat HIV and AIDS.

The Blair government in Britain is doing great work to raise the profile of diseases of the brain. The government recently committed more than $1.5 billion in new funding for research and treatment of mental illness. In establishing goals for the national health care system, the government gave mental illness top priority, alongside coronary heart disease. The government has established clear benchmarks of success, such as a 20-per-cent drop in the national suicide rate within a decade.

In the United States, the first-ever White House Conference on Mental Health in 1999 called for a national anti-stigma campaign. And the first-ever Surgeon General's Report on Mental Health noted that nearly half of all Americans who have a severe mental illness do not seek treatment. Most often, the reluctance to seek care is a direct result of the stigma.

Great strides are being made in other countries, which only underscores how much more needs to be done here. The federal government should embrace this issue as a top priority, just as other nations have done. As well as raising public understanding and awareness, the government should provide a level of research funding that acknowledges the scope and severity of these diseases.

We have nowhere near the proper level of funding. Research into schizophrenia, depression, and other psychiatric disorders has been maintained at a paltry level compared to other major disease groups, such as cancer, heart disease, stroke, AIDS, or Alzheimer's. Real progress in understanding illnesses of the brain will only come if funding is brought up to the level available for the study of these other diseases. There is simply no excuse for the meagre number of research dollars currently made available.

Government funding suffers from the stigma. The false assumptions that are always made about mental illness being a personal weakness have tainted government policy. Our political decision-makers simply don't believe that mental illnesses are as preventable, treatable, or curable, as are diseases that attack other parts of the body. But they are. And since these illnesses arise from dysfunction of the most complicated part of the human body – the brain – enormous research efforts will be required to advance our knowledge.

Stigmas are founded on ignorance. The antidote for ignorance is knowledge. In the last few years, the most important tool ever for sharing knowledge and communicating has thundered onto the scene. The Internet can deal a powerful blow to stigma.

In one stellar example of what can be done, a number of individuals and companies came together to create the international Open the Doors campaign in concert with the World Psychiatric Association.

So far, the program to fight the stigma and discrimination associated with schizophrenia has been initiated in fourteen countries, including Canada.

A key component of the six-year-old program is the Web site <www.openthedoors.com>, where participants can access the truth. Measurable results have been achieved in countries where the program was tested. In Canada, these results included changing admission procedures for emergency rooms nationally, and changes in knowledge and attitudes among high school students.

This is a great initiative in harnessing the power of the Net.

I'm an admirer of the French novelist and philosopher Victor Hugo, who said there is nothing so powerful as an idea whose time has come. Perhaps the time has finally come for a fundamental change in public attitudes about brain disorders. The time has come for another $12 million and $120 million and $1.2 billion to give the resources our brilliant researchers urgently need to understand the real causes of illness and develop truly effective prevention and treatment programs. And hopefully the time has come for each of us to redouble our energies to make that future scenario a reality for the young Daves of the world.

Don Tapscott is an entrepreneur, consultant, and author of several books on business, the Internet, and new technologies. Vice-President Al Gore has called him one of the world's leading "cyber-gurus." This article is adapted from an address given to the Canadian Psychiatric Research Foundation in December 2000.

"A CALL TO ARMS: PART TWO"

There is one more vision we'd like to share – a parting "call to arms" that we believe perfectly complements Don Tapscott's passionate call for funding and research. In fact, it's the other side of the same coin.

It's a vision we stressed throughout *The Last Taboo*, one we believe in so strongly, we feel compelled to write about it here. It's a vision that's shared by a man named William Anthony. He's the executive director of a research and training facility at Boston University known as the Center for Psychiatric Rehabilitation. He was kind enough, despite a busy schedule, to sit down for a coffee with us during a recent trip to Canada.

A clinical psychologist by trade, Dr. Anthony is something of a visionary in the field of mental health. To grossly oversimplify things, he's considered one of the world's leading experts on resilience and recovery, on the supports that people with mental illness say they need to get well and stay well. He's devoted his life to the field.

In fact, many years before we started writing books, Anthony and his colleagues were paying attention to the same kinds of stories. Back in the 1970s, Anthony and a few other progressive thinkers began doing something extremely unorthodox. They began *listening* to people struggling with mental illness – listening to the hopes, dreams, frustrations, and anger of ordinary people coping with extraordinary challenges.

Then they took things a logical step further.

"We started asking people what they *wanted*. Nobody had done that in the past. People with psychiatric disabilities had not been asked what they wanted or needed," he said during a speech to the International Association of Psycho Social Rehabilitation Services.

The reason no one had been asking was because of a long-standing and, at the time, virtually unchallenged assumption: that individuals with mental illness were damaged, flawed people who would never recover and, in most cases, certainly did not know what was best for them. In that era, the widespread perception was that the most optimistic outcome one could hope for was simply to *maintain* these folks – to keep them "stable."

Once Anthony started asking questions, however, he began hearing what were at the time pretty startling answers. People said they were capable of – indeed, they craved – far more.

"We found out that people were much more than their impairments, much more than their diagnoses, which is the way we, as a field, were treating folks at that time," he says.

In those days, it was easy to view someone simply as "a schizophrenic," or "a manic-depressive." Anthony looked beyond the label. He put on a wide-angle lens and focused on the whole person. It may not seem quite so radical now, but it most certainly was then.

"We looked at the fact that skills and symptoms weren't related – that if you knew only about a person's symptoms, you didn't know about that person's dreams and goals and skills and desires. You had just a partial picture of that person," he told us.

It wasn't the same kind of research as examining serotonin levels in people with depression, and Anthony's data was initially criticized by some as being too "soft," too subjective. But he believes, as we do, that it is infused with meaning.

"To me, we can learn as much from the narrative and the story as we can from some of the objective research," he explains.

After decades in the field, Anthony has come to believe very deeply that we need to change the way our mental health services are delivered – that we must base our systems, our perceptions, our supports on what people say they need to recover from a catastrophe. Not merely from the *symptoms* of mental illness, but from the far wider catastrophe of being mentally ill.

To demonstrate, Anthony did a pretty neat thing during that recent Canadian speech. He asked audience members to recall a catastrophe that had occurred in their lives. Perhaps it was a death in the family, a serious physical injury, a divorce. It could be any kind of catastrophe or trauma as long as it was not an episode of mental illness.

He then asked folks to describe, in a single word, how they felt at the time.

"Anxious!" shouted one woman. "Desperate!" chimed in someone sitting next to her. Soon, there was a chorus of words to describe terrible periods in the audience's lives. Words like "lonely" and "isolated," or "angry" and "trapped." Anthony repeated each word. He then posed an intriguing question.

"What if that had been a *mental* health catastrophe?" he asked. "What would clinicians say about those feelings?"

He stopped for a moment, then delivered a potential answer that spoke volumes. "They'd say, 'That's just part of your diagnosis – you trapped, desperate, confused, isolated, anxiety-ridden person, you.'"

Anthony let that sink in, really sink in. He then continued with an observation.

"We're approaching this whole field of mental health recovery far too simplistically. We have to pay attention to these feelings. These are *normal* responses to a catastrophe. And being labelled and diagnosed and treated for a mental illness is a catastrophe. It *is* a catastrophe. But it is also something that people can move through and find new meaning and growth in their lives."

And how, precisely, do they do that?

"When I asked people what helped them recover, they talked about people who believed in them. About work, hope, talking, reading, hugging – all these other things that are not necessarily medication and therapy." In other words, the same things we all need when we're struggling through life.

Problem is, says Anthony (or, more accurately, people have repeatedly *told* Anthony), our mental health systems are rarely responsive to those needs.

"Unfortunately, our whole system was designed on, and has practised for a hundred years, a non-recovery model. So all of our training programs, our funding incentives, and so forth, are set up to believe that recovery is not possible."

It's important to note that William Anthony is not opposed to medication, or the doctors who prescribe it. "People who have recovered are still using medication," he says. "This is not an anti-medication, anti-medical-model direction. It's saying that the people who are delivering the meds really need to understand that they're treating the whole person. Not just a disease, not just a symptom. They have to put it in the context of meaning and purpose in a person's life."

In fact, Anthony's goal is one we believe *all* mental health professionals can share. "What I've tried to say that people can agree on is recovery. You can have doctors prescribing medication in the service of recovery, and you can have people who take a psycho social approach doing rehab in the service of recovery. The recovery itself transcends all these disciplines, services, and labels."

When we started writing this book, our original goal was simple: we hoped to take a big whack at stigma. To show that mental illness hits all kinds of people, and for all kinds of reasons. And to show that people can, and do, recover in all kinds of ways. It's a message we hope will reach people who know nothing about mental illness, as well as people who know it intimately – those now struggling towards recovery, and those who love them.

"People *can* recover," William Anthony stresses. "Most of the people who have recovered have been at the depths of depression or the depths of some other illness, and they have made it back to find a life worth living with meaning and purpose. I think that's the story that only people who've been there can give. I can say it, but I can't say it quite like somebody who's lived it."

Throughout this book, we've tried to let the people who *have* lived it tell us their own stories. In writing these closing pages, it dawned on us that many of the themes and messages that kept surfacing are the same ones William A. Anthony has been hearing – and writing about – for many years. Needs that, at their core, are exceedingly human.

It leaves us with mixed feelings, this realization.

After decades of work by Anthony and others, it is frustrating to know that the same themes and messages still need to be spread.

But there is satisfaction, too, in knowing that more and more people are willing to talk – by speaking out about their experiences, their needs, what helps them, what doesn't. By sharing their stories here, we are simply trying to help spread the word. To help spread *their* words.

Praise for *The Last Taboo*
(now available in paperback)

"The best . . . book ever written about mental illness and mental health in Canada."　　　　　– Canadian Mental Health Association

"I know of only a few books that explain mental health and illness well to the general reader. *The Last Taboo* is now one of these books, and it gives a welcome Canadian perspective. . . . It is well-written and entertaining."　　　　　　　　　　　– Montreal *Gazette*

"Solid research and a harrowing personal story."
　　　　　　　　　　　　　　　　　– Halifax *Daily News*

"There is more learning and plain talk . . . within the pages of this book than most of us have found in lifetimes spent in doctor's offices and psychiatric wards. *The Last Taboo* renews hope in those who've despaired over closed doors and closed minds."
　　　　　– Pat Capponi, author of *Upstairs in the Crazy House*

"An important book that deserves wide readership."
　　　　　　　　　　　　　　　　　　– *Edmonton Journal*

"A guide to everything from the role of genetics, the environment and the law to current therapies, drugs, and alternative treatments. It offers the hope that recovery is possible."
　　　　　　　　　　　– Pamela Wallin, Globebooks.com

"A most helpful tour of the mental health system thickets . . . a road map and travellers' tale all in one."　　　　　– *Toronto Star*

"*The Last Taboo* addresses a topic that has been crying out for such a carefully crafted, well-reasoned, and optimistic treatment. It is a unique blend of useful information, personal insights, and superior storytelling . . . a hopeful book . . . and an encouragement to all of us living and working in the field."
　　　　　　　　　　　– William A. Anthony, Executive Director,
　　　　　　　　　　　Boston Center for Psychiatric Rehabilitation

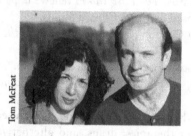

Tom McFeat

Julia Nunes has worked in journalism for fifteen years, as an arts reporter for the *Globe and Mail*, a news reporter and writer/editor for CBC Television, and as a radio producer and reporter. She has lived and worked in several Canadian cities, and in London, Prague, and Moscow. She currently produces science documentaries for the Discovery Channel.

Scott Simmie is a columnist for the *Toronto Star* with more than 21 years' experience as a journalist in radio, print, and television. He has worked over the years in China, London, Thailand, and Russia. In 1989 he reported on the Chinese democracy movement for the CBC, and later that year co-authored the critically acclaimed book *Tiananmen Square*.